W9-COD-533

DEMCO

Claude A. Frazier, M.D., is one of America's leading authorities on allergies. He is certified in both allergy and pediatrics and is a Fellow of the American Academy of Pediatrics, the American Academy of Allergy, and the American College of Allergists. Every year Dr. Frazier edits the *Annual Review of Allergy*.

COPING & LIVING WITH ALLERGIES

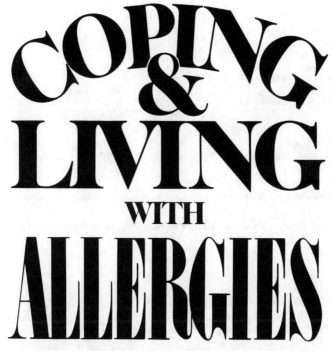

COPING & LIVING WITH ALLERGIES

A COMPLETE GUIDE TO HELP ALLERGY PATIENTS OF ALL AGES

Claude A. Frazier, M.D.

A SPECTRUM BOOK

PRENTICE-HALL, INC., *Englewood Cliffs, New Jersey 07632*

Library of Congress Cataloging in Publication Data

Frazier, Claude Albee, 1920–
　Coping & living with allergies.

　(A Spectrum Book)
　Bibliography: p.
　Includes index.
　1. Allergy. I. Title.
RC584.F68　　616.97　　80–18552
ISBN　0-13-172304-9
ISBN　0-13-172296-4 (pbk.)

Editorial production/supervision and interior design
　by *Heath Lynn Silberfeld*
Manufacturing buyer: *Cathie Lenard*
Cover design by *Honi Werner*

10　9　8　7　6　5　4　3　2　1

Printed in the United States of America

PRENTICE-HALL INTERNATIONAL, INC., *London*
PRENTICE-HALL OF AUSTRALIA PTY. LIMITED, *Sydney*
PRENTICE-HALL OF CANADA, LTD., *Toronto*
PRENTICE-HALL OF INDIA PRIVATE LIMITED, *New Delhi*
PRENTICE-HALL OF JAPAN, INC., *Tokyo*
PRENTICE-HALL OF SOUTHEAST ASIA PTE. LTD., *Singapore*
WHITEHALL BOOKS LIMITED, *Wellington, New Zealand*

Contents

Lucretius, Roman poet and philosopher who lived in the first century before Christ, said, "What is food to one, is to others bitter poison." This could well have been his epitaph, for it is said that he committed suicide in a fit of madness induced by a love potion fed to him by his wife.

This very old adage can be aptly applied to allergy, for what is harmless and well tolerated by most people can make the allergic ill, sometimes very ill. It is this uniqueness of some individuals that has made allergy a somewhat mysterious disease, and those who are unaffected by its various miseries are inclined to attribute its symptoms as being mainly "in the head" of the victims. Actually, allergy is a far more common health problem in the United States than either the public or the medical profession realizes. And it may be an increasing health problem, for we are introducing new substances into our environment almost daily. Some of these chemicals have never been seen in nature before; therefore, we may not have time to adapt to them, nor may we be able to easily. Some of these substances are toxic and bitter poison to us all. Many, however, are allergenic and bitter poison only for the hypersensi-

Preface

tive, the allergic. Considering that perhaps one in four or one in five Americans is allergic to something inhaled, ingested, contacted, or injected into the body, it is high time we understood this strange and very complex disease. For allergy is a disease. It does not reside within its victim's head. The allergic are not simply neurotic or hypochondrial. They are ill, and their illness is often chronic, sometimes temporary, and sometimes, fortunately somewhat rarely, fatal. And never very comfortable!

CLAUDE A. FRAZIER, M.D.

I would like to express my appreciation to *Frieda K. Brown*, without whose help this book would not have been a reality.

COPING & LIVING WITH ALLERGIES

PART I

ALLERGY: HOW IT WORKS

one

From the heart of this fountain of delight wells up some bitter taste to choke them even amid the flowers.

Lucretius

As the reader can surmise, I am fond of Lucretius. And here again he could be speaking of allergy. Those unfortunates who choke amid the flowers could be responding to some nearby ragweed. Or the bitter taste could be caused by an allergic reaction to a glass of perfectly good cow's milk. It is the normally harmless, the usually very ordinary, things contacted every day which can produce symptoms of illness for the hypersensitive. This is the crux of the definition of allergy, that it is an altered response to substances which ordinarily have no harmful effect on the majority of people.

Somewhere in the neighborhood of 30 million Americans suffer from some form of allergy in reaction to something they inhale or ingest or contact or are injected with, and their symptoms range from being so mild as to be scarcely noticeable to so severe as to be fatal. They may suffer seasonal bouts

Things Are Not What They Seem

with allergies or be chronically ill the year around, depending on what in their environment generates their overreaction. Unfortunately for them, since almost everyone else around them tolerates whatever it is that is making them ill, they often find themselves openly or silently accused of being neurotic or hypochondrial. After all, how can anyone be poisoned by something essentially nontoxic, usually quite ordinary, and often delicious or very pleasant? The lot of the allergic individual is to be frequently misunderstood and as frequently dismissed as someone lacking in intestinal fortitude.

Recognition of allergy as a disease entity is only a little over half a century old. In spite of Lucretius and the efforts of a nineteenth-century physician, Charles H. Blackley, who wrote of his own rhinitis, which he deduced was caused by exposure to grass pollen, allergy is a relatively young medical specialty. Endowed with a scientist's curiosity, Blackley applied grass pollen to his own skin and was rewarded by a hivelike eruption. On this odd response, he built a detailed study, the first real attempt to comprehend the hypersensitivity phenomenon. Alas, his meticulous monograph gathered dust for many years, until researchers became interested in the problems of immunology and in the development of various immunizing techniques such as antitoxin for diphtheria.

In France, meanwhile, Charles Richet noted several phenomena which he labeled anaphylaxis. He observed that an initial injection of a foreign substance might cause no adverse effects in some individuals, but that a reinjection of the same material could cause strange, even severe symptoms of illness. He also noticed that to produce such a response a time lapse, generally of several days, appeared necessary between injections.

Later pioneers in their studies of such altered responses broadened their views to include far more frequent and milder reactions than anaphylaxis, which they called allergic responses in contrast to the more violent anaphylactic reaction. Around the turn of the century Clement Von Pirquet coined the word *allergy* when he discovered that patients who recovered from a bout with tuberculosis reacted positively to a skin test with tuberculin organisms. Studies of experimental anaphylaxis with laboratory animals soon became correlated with hypersensitivity (allergic) reactions in humans, and the discipline of allergy was off and running. Recent studies in immunology have greatly facilitated the understanding of the allergic response; thus, to penetrate the mysteries of allergy, we should first understand a bit about this larger subject.

Time was when the immune process was considered as being only beneficial, conferring protection for us against bacteria, combating infection.

However, we now know that this whole process can also be harmful, for allergic reactions are essentially immune responses, although somewhat overblown. We can say that they are overreactions of the body's defense system against the invasion of what the body considers foreign. The word *immunity* was derived from the Latin word meaning "to free of burden," but such a meaning no longer really fits our modern concept of the process, for it may impose a burden on some people as well as lift one.

In his book *Immunology*, Dr. Joseph A. Bellanti has defined immunity as "all those physiologic mechanisms which endow the animal with the capacity to recognize materials as foreign to itself and to neutralize, eliminate or metabolize them with or without injury to its own tissues." Allergy, of course, occurs because this process does injure the hypersensitive person's tissues. The word *antigen* is used to designate such foreign materials; when speaking of antigens which produce the altered response of allergy, we frequently discriminate from other antigens such as bacteria with the word *allergen.* In general, antigens can produce either beneficial or harmful responses, whereas allergens produce the harmful response of allergy. Allergens are commonly of heavy molecular weight, with proteins as the chief villains, although some polysaccharides (two types of carbohydrates—starches and cellulose) of considerable molecular weight can also provoke allergic reactions.

Allergens, however, are not the only culprits. Certain simple chemical compounds, which in themselves are not capable of eliciting an allergic response, have a nasty habit of combining with a protein, often one of the individual's own body proteins, to become an antigen that is capable of producing symptoms of allergy. These are called *haptens,* and their discovery has shed light on some of allergy's more mysterious facets.

The animal embryo does not start out possessing protection against antigens, and every once in a blue moon an infant is born without an immune system. Such children are kept alive only in a completely sterile environment such as that enclosing David, the boy in the plastic bubble. (David, incidentally, now eight, has slowly been assembling bits and pieces of an immune system through the years, and researchers have learned a great deal from his predicament.) In the early stages of the embryo's development, tissue from another organism can be transplanted without rejection. Oddly enough, when the animal that has had such tissue transplanted into its own tissue as an embryo receives a second transplant later in life from the same organism, the transplant will once again be accepted. Past this initial imunity-free stage, however, an elaborate protective system is developed to guard certain target cells in the various systems of our bodies—gastrointestinal tract, respiratory and circulatory systems, the skin and the central nervous system—from potential damage that could be initiated by substances foreign to the body and, sometimes, even from the body's own substances in what are called *autoimmune diseases.* We discuss the latter in a later chapter, for they present one of allergy's abiding mysteries.

Almost all living organisms possess a system for determining "self" from "nonself". Even a plant has a mechanism for separating pathogens from its own tissues. The immune system takes this recognition of self many steps further than the primitive models of plants and lower animal organisms, for it possesses a sort of memory which allows it to be specific in its selection of foreign substances to be repelled or neutralized. The first line of defense against infection are the phagocytes, cells which engulf, ingest, and eliminate such foreign intruders as bacteria. They stand at the ready on the body's battlements to ward off invasion, and if you are imaginative, you can think of them as soldier cells fully armed. Supporting them are mediator cells, which, on encountering an offending foreign agent, release chemical substances such as histamine, serotonin, and bradykinin. It is these mediators that actually cause tissue and organ damage. Histamine lowers blood pressure and increases gastric secretions. It contracts smooth muscles, such as are wrapped around the bronchi, and dilates blood vessels. Serotonin, on the other hand, constricts large blood vessels and contracts some smooth muscles. By and large, its role in allergy is not considered very important. The kinins are still something of a mystery, and it is questionable whether they are products of the antibody-antigen clash or of the tissue damage that results. It is known that they can contract smooth muscle, cause pain, and dilate blood vessels and increase their permeability. Another mediator called SRS-A (slow-reacting substance) has been implicated in bronchoconstriction in asthma.

To simplify what is exceedingly complex, an allergen enters the body and reacts with an antibody (reagin) fixed to the surface of certain cells called *mast cells.* When the antibody binds the allergen, it triggers the release of the mediators. The mediators apparently cause the symptoms of allergy through their mechanisms of contracting smooth muscle, dilating blood vessels, increasing the permeability of blood vessels so that there is a leakage of fluid, and stimulating mucous glands to produce increased quantities of mucus. The part of the body affected in this process depends on whether the allergen was inhaled, ingested, injected, or contacted and which system or organ of the body has antibody-carrying mast cells in abundance. The latter is called the shock organ. In essence, it receives the brunt of the antibody-allergen clash.

Our bodies manufacture a variety of antibodies, called *immunoglobulins.*

There are five identifiable types which we can, fortunately, shorten to Ig's: IgG, IgE, IgA, IgM, and IgD. IgE is the immunoglobulin associated with allergy and the one, therefore, that we deal with, because the allergic individual, perhaps because of a genetic predisposition, tends to overproduce this particular antibody in an altered response to allergenic substances. We all possess IgE, with the exception of those who are immune deficient; in fact, we all could become allergic to something at some time in our lives if conditions were favorable for sensitization.

Increased production of IgE is part and parcel of the mechanism of sensitization. The susceptible individual must first be exposed to an allergen to bring about this increase, which, on subsequent exposures to the same allergen, brings on the antibody-allergen clash. This is sensitization. Sensitization can occur in a single exposure, or it may take repeated exposures before an allergic reaction occurs. For example, an individual may be stung by a honeybee, and his reaction may be quite mild and normal; however, on being restung several months later, he may suffer life-threatening anaphylactic shock. Another individual fighting off an infection might have repeated injections of penicillin before suddenly reacting with symptoms of allergy.

A number of factors play a role in the development of allergy. Perhaps the strongest is that of genetic predisposition. If allergy runs in one side of a person's family, that person has about a 50% chance of developing an allergy himself. If it runs in both sides, the chances for the person being allergic to something increases to around 75%. The allergy diseases may not be the same as those of one's forebears, nor may the allergens one is hypersensitive to be those of one's relatives.

The nature of the allergen itself and the amount and duration of exposure are important factors in sensitization. Some allergens are potent sensitizers. Penicillin and poison ivy are excellent examples. Sometimes repeated exposure over a period of time results in the development of sensitivity to an allergen. People who live surrounded by ragweed may eventually develop hay fever, particularly if their inheritance is such to predispose them to allergy.

Infection plays a major role in the development of allergy, and vice versa. A person suffering an upper-respiratory illness who is predisposed to allergy may move from the infection into symptoms of allergy, such as perennial rhinitis or asthma. The general theory has been that infective agents act as stimuli, lowering the allergically predisposed individual's tolerance level to allergens, but more recently it has been suggested that such patients may be reacting allergically to the infective agent itself.

Oddly enough, weather change and temperature may also be factors in allergy. Sudden barometric rises or falls or abrupt changes in temperature may act as triggers for allergic diseases, especially for asthma.

Emotional stress plays an ambiguous role, especially in asthma and gastrointestinal allergy. It is an equivocal factor, because it may be a trigger for allergy or it may be a result of allergy, and deciding whether it precedes or follows is very much a chicken versus egg question. There is no doubt that the physical alterations stress can make in the body can precipitate allergy diseases. Equally, there is no doubt that some allergy diseases such as asthma and eczema create emotional stress, which can then aggravate allergy symptoms. Cause and effect in this area remains a bit murky.

Although there is some uncertainty as to the role of these various factors in the production of allergy symptoms, we do know that sensitization itself requires an initial exposure to an allergen or allergens and that a given time lapse must occur between this initial exposure and a second contact with the allergen. During this period, IgE antibodies specific for that particular allergen are produced in the blood and circulated to various body tissues. In some of these tissues, say, in the respiratory system, they become bound to the mast cells residing in body connective tissues, usually in close proximity to the mucous membranes of the respiratory and gastrointestinal tracts. These are target cells and contain histamine and the other mediators mentioned earlier. When the foreign allergen once again invades, these cells release histamine, and the other mediators as their adhering antibodies do battle and bind the invading allergen, now clearly recognized as the enemy. As we have noted, it is the mediators, histamine chiefly, released in this antibody-allergen clash that do the actual damage to body tissues. Smooth muscles around the bronchi may contract to cause airway obstruction; mucous membranes may swell to increase that obstruction, and mucous glands may produce an overabundance of mucus to further complicate matters. Blood vessels may dilate and thin so that they leak fluid into tissues to cause edema.

The strange part about all this is the specificity of this process, for the IgE antibody with receptors specially designed to bind ragweed pollen allergens may pay no attention to other allergenic substances that come down the pike. However, a person may be hypersensitive to more than one allergenic substance. In fact, there are some unfortunate people who seem to be allergic to almost everthing in the environment. Newspapers delight in finding such an individual and detailing all the normal activities he cannot participate in without becoming ill. Fortunately, such all-encompassing allergy is rare. However, a cross-reaction to allergens somewhat similar in their components to the allergen responsible for the original sensitization is not rare. An individual allergic to peanuts, for instance, may also find himself allergic to peas, for these two common foods belong to the same botanical family and are thus somewhat similar in their composition.

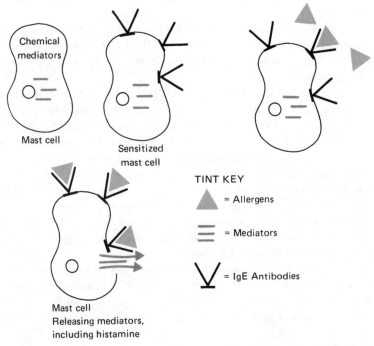

The process of sensitization.

For ease of description, let us follow Dr. Bellanti's lead and divide the immunological process into three stages, although we are discussing allergy and allergens, whereas his discussion dealt with antigens, which includes allergens as well as bacteria and viruses. The first or primary stage consists of the elimination of the antigen by the process of phagocytosis, the digestion of the substances foreign to the body by the defending phagocyte cells. If the antigen escapes this first line of defense and persists, a secondary process occurs in which antibodies specific to that antigen are developed with memory cells that will recognize it when they meet again. Generally, the antigen is eliminated at this stage, but if it still persists, either because of its somewhat indestructible nature or because the invaded host possesses a genetic weakness of the immunological system, four types of deleterious responses may occur.

Type I is an immediate (allergic) response mediated by IgE antibodies. Types II and III produce disease outside the scope of this book, and Type IV produces symptoms of a delayed hypersensitivity reaction like that seen in contact dermatitis to such substances as poison ivy or to certain metals such as nickel.

As we have noted earlier, there are substances, commonly simple chemicals which, although nonallergenic in themselves, combine with proteins, generally those furnished by the body of the host, to form haptens capable of causing sensitization.

By now the reader must be aware that allergy is a complex subject and that I have barely skimmed the surface. Annually new hypotheses are proposed to shift the substance of our knowledge, and new findings are piled on old. And in the meantime, allergy is apparently on the increase among modern populations, no doubt because of an ever-increasing use of new chemicals and the widespread pollution of the air, water, and foodstuffs. Since our species has never encountered some of these substances, we have had no chance to adapt physically to their presence in our technological world (nor, perhaps, mentally either). We have also drastically altered the natural world, replacing, for instance, the forests with highways, homes, and shopping centers. Such riotous plants as ragweed have taken full advantage of the disturbed ecology and have propagated in abundance wherever our mania for bulldozing the land has toppled the normal order of plant life. This has been unfortunate for many who react to the annual onslaught of ragweed pollen. It is doubtful that the caveman suffered from allergy, although I am sure that this would be a difficult statement to prove. Statistically, though, modern societies do sport greater incidences of allergy sufferers than do less complex groups, so it does seem to be a disease of the civilized.

GLOSSARY

Hypersensitivity: employed interchangeably with allergy. Describes allergic state.

Immunity: defined by Dr. Joseph A. Bellanti as "all those physiologic mechanisms which endow the animal with the capacity to recognize materials as foreign to itself and to neutralize, eliminate or metabolize them with or without injury to its own tissues."

Allergen: an antigen; usually a protein of high molecular weight.

Hapten: a substance not allergenic in itself but capable of producing allergy disease when it combines with some proteins.

Autoimmune disease: symptoms caused by the body's immune reaction to its own products.

Phagocytes: cells which engulf, ingest, and eliminate foreign substances.

Mediators: substances—histamine, for example—contained in mast cells and basophiles.

Mast cells: connective tissue cells important for their cellular defense mechanism during injury or infection.

Basophile: a white blood cell.

Immunoglobulins: antibodies. Protein substances developed usually in response to the presence of an antigen.

SUMMARY

1. Allergy can be defined as an abnormal response to substances well tolerated by most people. It is part of the immune process.

2. An allergen is an antigen or agent capable of producing symptoms of allergy.

3. Prior exposure to an allergen is necessary to produce sensitization in the susceptible individual. Once sensitized, the allergic person may then exhibit an altered response when exposed again to that specific allergen.

4. It is probable that anyone could be made allergic to something under the proper conditions of exposure. However, heredity, the amount and duration of exposure to a given allergen, and the nature and potency of that allergen are major factors in determining who will suffer allergy disease.

5. Immunoglobulin E (IgE) is the antibody associated with an allergic reaction.

6. There are two main types of allergic reactions—immediate and delayed.

two

We exist in an environment which is benign for the most part, but like everything else in life, there are exceptions, little imperfections to spoil our enjoyment. For an estimated 20% of the population of the United States, one group of Nature's flaws, allergens, can be all important to health and happiness, although those of us untouched by such strangeness may wonder why perfectly normal substances should make anyone ill. In fact, we might well doubt their existence, for these substances are, after all, the stuff of life. This makes it very difficult for the one in five people who is hypersensitive. The healthy among us are likely to burden them with blame for their vulnerability to everyday things. For we must remember that when we speak of allergens, we are talking generally about perfectly natural substances—not toxic, not infectious, not contagious.

As we have noted, allergens are usually proteins of high molecular weight, although some members of the carbohydrate family, the polysaccharides, may also contain allergens. We have defined an allergen as a substance which induces an antibody response to produce an allergic reaction

Allergens at Work

in the susceptible individual. We noted that the havoc a specific allergen can cause depends on a number of variables, including the amount, duration, and route of exposure. The extent of such reactions also varies from individual to individual.

Almost anything can happen when allergens and the allergic get together, for just about every body system or organ can register symptoms of an allergic reaction, ranging from discomfort to disability. In addition, and this is often as difficult for a physician to understand as for a layperson, allergy symptoms in a specific body system may be accompanied by general feelings of malaise, of plain not feeling up to scratch, of being out of sorts, out of kilter. For example, frequently an asthma patient suffers emotional disturbances which, in part, may arise from the stress of his disease but which also may be caused by an allergic reaction occurring in his central nervous system. On the other hand, an allergic reaction in the central nervous system may produce these feelings without a specific symptom for either physician or patient to put a finger on.

Because symptoms of allergy are similar to those of other diseases, some of them serious indeed, the physician must rule them out before he can rule allergy in. Generally, he or she begins the diagnostic process by taking a thorough patient history. This initial step is important in any medical diagnosis, but it is especially so in allergy. The history is a kind of compendium of the patient's life and includes what he or she eats, breathes, takes as medication, does to earn a living, lives in, has as a life-style, and so on. Even the family relationships are included, plus health problems of parents, siblings, and any children, since allergy is considered an inherited predisposition. The time of year symptoms occur and whether they are worse in evenings and better in mornings are all significant questions. Ascertaining whether a cat, dog, or other furry pet lives in the home may be just as significant, as can questions about what sort of pillows, blankets, and mattresses are used and even how old they are, for aging overstuffed furniture and mattresses can become potently allergenic, and feather pillows have caused a good deal of misery in their time for the hypersensitive. Hobbies and how the home is heated are also germane.

An impatient patient eager to get to the root of the trouble may become somewhat restless during this grilling and even consider the physician's questioning not only irrelevant but highly personal. The patient should realize that every question has its reasons and that somewhere in the answers lie clues as to what allergens in the environment are causing the illness. For example, if the patient suffers symptoms of rhinitis only in the spring, an allergy to tree or grass pollens may be suspected. It will probably be tree pollen if symptoms are present early in the spring from February to June, depending, of course, on the locale and the species that are present. Grass pollinates somewhat later, usually from about the middle of May until early July, again depending upon the locale and the species. In either case, when symptoms appear is important in determining the allergen at work. Or if the patient appears to be affected during the work week but is relatively symptom-free on weekends, the chances are good that exposure to some allergen connected with employment is at the root of the problem. Incidentally, occupational allergy appears to be on the increase.

Although the patient's history will provide a major part of the diagnostic story, the physician will wish to conduct a thorough physical examination, followed probably by a number of laboratory tests, perhaps including some X-rays. When other possibilities for the patient's symptoms can be discarded, the physician can turn full attention to the probability of allergy. It now becomes a hunt for the offending allergen or allergens.

If inhalant allergens such as pollens, for instance, are suspected, skin tests or the new RAST test will be given. Though not 100% reliable (little in medicine is), skin testing, properly done, is probably the most determinate of the two. Both types of tests commonly serve to pinpoint the specific allergen or allergens causing the problem, as well as some degree of the patient's hypersensitivity level. Skin tests are not reliable in the case of allergy to food, with the exception of food allergens producing an immediate and usually severe reaction. In this latter case it then becomes too dangerous to employ skin tests, since a severe, evern life-threatening response could be induced. In any case, when this kind of reaction is experienced both the physician and the patient are almost always well aware of the cause. In less dramatic and drastic allergic reactions to food, the only really sure way to unmask the offending allergens is to employ an elimination diet, which we discuss in a later chapter. Suffice it to say here that the diet lives up to its name by eliminating a good part of the patient's ordinary fare, invariably what is liked most and is fun and fattening. Once the patient is on a bare-bones sort of menu, foods are reintroduced one by one to see which item of diet is the culprit and produces the symptoms.

The patient's history with its detailed questions plus the location and appearance of lesions on the skin often are enough to make a case against allergens producing contact dermatitis. However, when in doubt, the physician may challenge the patient's hide by patch testing, a procedure in which the suspected allergen is applied in proper concentrations to the skin via a patch of gauze or Band-Aid and allowed to stay in contact for a sufficient period to produce results, usually 24 to 48 hours. If the suspected offending agent is an irritant, however, it should not be employed in patch testing, since it can cause considerable harm to the skin as well as produce allergic dermatitis.

Skin tests have long been one of the most useful tools in the allergist's stock in trade. These tests come in four forms: scratch, prick, intradermal, and passive transfer. Scratch and prick tests are just that—a tiny scratch or prick is made in the skin, usually on the back or inner arm below the elbow, and a drop of an extract of the allergen to be tested is rubbed into the minute break. The patient then sits comfortably in the office or waiting room for at least 20 minutes, time enough to allow an allergic reaction (very minor) to make itself known if it is going to occur. If nothing shows up at the site of scratch or prick, the test is considered negative. However, the patient cannot yet be considered in the clear in regard to this particular allergen, for it is possible that the extract employed was too weak to provoke a reaction. The physician may resort to a stronger extract or turn to intradermal testing, which consists of injecting a tiny amount of the extract just beneath the skin. Generally, the intradermal test is more certain to detect mild hypersensitivity that a scratch test can miss. However, since it can also produce a severe reaction in a patient whose hypersensitivity is potent, it is generally not employed when the patient's history suggests such a reaction is possible.

Usually a positive result in skin testing is no more than a small red spot or wheal much like a mosquito bite at the site of scratch, prick, or injection. It may be accompanied by a slight swelling and/or a little itching. The size of the wheal and whether it has pseudopods (false feet) indicate to some extent the strength of the patient's hypersensitivity. And since there is always the possibility that a patient may react with severe, generalized symptoms to skin tests, the physician wisely begins with weak extracts and works up to more potent solutions, depending on the initial results. Coming on too strong in the physician's office can be as unfortunate as at a cocktail party or in a new job!

Passive transfer testing is occasionally employed when the physician suspects that the reaction to even a weak extract might be hazardous or if the patient's skin is in such bad shape from widespread eczema or hives that adding insult to injury is not advisable. A bit of the patient's blood is withdrawn instead and transferred to the skin of a person known to be nonallergic, preferably of no relation to the patient. Skin tests are then performed on the recipient of the patient's blood, who would respond as the patient would, since he or she now possesses the patient's antibodies. At least, ideally, this occurs. There are problems with passive transfer, the main one being the possibility of transferring hepatitis.

A recent method of pursuing allergens has been developed. Called RAST (a happy shortening of radioallergosorbent test, an uncomfortable mouthful, even for a physician), it is shiny and modern and at ease in our technological society. Even so, many allergists still prefer to employ it in conjunction with skin tests rather than rely totally on it, for its development is so new that we are not yet certain about its accuracy in all situations. Because it is *in vitro* (done apart from the body, as in a test tube), it has definite advantages, but it is also fiercely expensive at present and uncommonly complex; thus it may not be an ideal office procedure for the average physician or even for the everyday allergist. Worse still, so far it has proved to be about 80% as accurate as skin testing.

Still, it is an interesting development and may yet prove vital in the specialty of allergy. The description I offer here sadly lacks the complexity of the procedure itself, but it will have to do in place of a trip to the laboratory and a step-by-step runthrough of the RAST process. A small amount of the patient's serum is removed, and a drop or so is married to the suspected allergen on a paper disk. This is then incubated for a few hours at room temperature, then washed to get rid of proteins not bound to the allergen. This procedure leaves the patient's antibodies that are specifically directed toward the allergen being tested. To estimate the strength or abundance of these IgE antibodies (the reader will remember that in Chapter 1 we noted that IgE antibodies are produced in more than normal quantities by the allergic individual in response to an allergen to which he has become sensitized), anti-antibodies, if we can call them that to simplify matters, are added (to up the ante, you could say), and the whole is incubated again for a period of time, then washed to rid the disk of free anti-IgE antibodies. The remainder is then measured for radioactivity. The higher the count registered, the more IgE antibodies are bound to the allergen. Measurements have been worked out so that the physician can assess the relative strength of the patient's hypersensitivity.

I am glad that I began this description by warning that the procedure is complex, and I will understand completely if the reader is now heaving a sigh of relief. RAST is, I believe, one more example of where modern medicine has gone—sunk, it would seem, far from the nonmedical individual's sight into that spotless, glittering aluminum-glass-and-plastic world of technology. Even an ordinary practicing physician like me has difficulty following the mechanics of the new and exciting, much less judging the efficacy of such extravagant and wonderful breakthroughs. I think, however, it is safe to say, what with the expense and complexity of RAST, that for the forseeable future most allergic patients will find that a careful history, a physical examination, and less-rarified laboratory and other tests, skin tests among them, will be their physician's diagnostic tools.

Now that the allergic reader knows what awaits at the physician/allergist's office, let us look at the havoc allergens have wrought to send him or her there in the first place. Let all readers beware, however, of unnecessarily taking these symptoms unto themselves, for the power of suggestion resides tenaciously in us all, as medical students know perhaps best of all.

If we start on the outside and work our way inward, we find that allergy often sets its brand on the human hide with such dismaying symptoms as eczema, urticaria, and dermatitis, plus a variety of less easily determinate bumps and blisters and rashes.

Eczema, which was once thought to be due simply to nerves and was even called neurodermatitis, is a mighty itch, with secondary symptoms of redness, oozing, and crusting, brought on in all probability as much by the uncontrollable need to scratch as by the actual physical condition of the skin. It is an ailment many a mother has met in her infant, but older children and adults as well may respond to allergens with these disconcerting symptoms. Such allergens are often foods, but since eczema frequently accompanies hay fever and asthma, the offending agent may also be an inhalant. Physicians have noted that about half the infants who develop colic during the first six months of life, then suffer eczema, go on to develop hay fever and possibly asthma later on. In fact, this relationship of symptoms has been so frequently observed that allergists have dubbed it the "allergic march" and have emphasized the importance of treating and controlling eczema in its early stages to halt the possibility of such a "march."

Urticaria, which is a fancy name for hives, are fairly familiar as red welts or wheals, often surrounded by red halos, which pop out suddenly on the skin, frequently for no apparent reason as far as the victim can see. They can itch like fury and even burn like fire. They can be very large, sometimes even a foot in diameter, or very small, as those due to heat tend to be. Hives may be localized in certain areas, especially in areas where clothing exerts pressure such as the waistline, or they may be widespread over the entire body. Commonly their survival is brief if bitter. They are a frequent occurrence in children and may signify nothing, but chronic hives which persist or reoccur over a period of weeks should prompt a visit to the doctor for a bit of tracking down.

In diagnosing a good crop of stubborn hives the physician must also consider such conditions as the presence of intestinal parasites, an overactive thyroid, emotional disturbances, and several other organic diseases. When he or she has narrowed things down to allergy, the first thing to be considered should be hypersensitivity to foods, drugs, or bacteria, because these are common causes. Among foods artificial colors appear to be a large factor, especially tartrazine, a yellow dye. Among drugs aspirin is a chief villain and is, by the way, closely related to tartrazine. Penicillin is high on the list of potently allergenic drugs.

Although urticaria can stand alone as a symptom, it often accompanies other indications of allergy and may even herald the onrush of a severe generalized or anaphylactic shock reaction.

Angioedema (giant hives) is a somewhat peculiar symptom of allergy. It may occur as a localized swelling of one area of the body, often the face and especially in the area of the eye or the lip, or it can include the entire body. An illustration of the latter is the woman who had to keep three different clothing sizes on hand to accommodate her fluctuating measurements occasioned by her allergy. I have also heard of a man so allergic to peanuts that he gained seven pounds on eating a single one. Ballooning in this fashion is probably rare, but surely worthy of note in medical literature! Angioedema, previously called angioneurotic edema and attributed also to nerves, is no joking matter if it occurs in the throat area, for such dramatic swelling of tissues can obstruct the airways and threaten suffocation. Nor, I am sure, are patients amused whose lips swell up like some dweller of the Ubangi region or whose vision is obscured by swollen eyes.

Finally, there are assorted rashes, itches, bumps, and blisters which most frequently signify an allergic reaction to something contacted. For example, some people are so exquisitely sensitive to nickel that they cannot tolerate a nickel-plated zipper, much less a nickel-plated watchband, without bursting forth at the point of contact with red rashes or lesions and a mighty itch. Since modern life, as we have noted earlier, is so full of a number of things never conceived by Mother Nature, the physician must often employ some pretty fancy detective work to track down the agents of contact dermatitis.

While we are still on the outside, we should consider the eye, for though frequently symptoms of allergy are exhibited by the eye in conjunction with other allergy symptoms such as hay fever, the eye alone can register an allergic reaction. Contact with some cosmetics, pollens, house dust, and animal dander may be at the root of allergy of the eye. Even the ingestion of some foods can bring on the itching, burning, red-eyed look of allergic conjunctivitis. Or the eyelids may swell in response to an insect sting or to a food or drug. Cosmetics and even fingernail polish can leave a red rash over the eyelids, the latter when the allergic lady touches her lids shortly after applying her favorite color. Inflammation, ulcers, and scaling of the eyes may result as an allergic reaction to bacteria, and the tear glands may be affected by an allergic reaction to cause "dry eye," although this is by no means a certain connection.

As we move within the body, we note that the respiratory system is frequently involved in allergy. Hay fever, or rose fever as it used to be commonly called, is so common a health problem that it is often treated somewhat humorously, but it is no fun for the victim. Nor, incidentally, has it anything to do with hay or roses, and it rarely sports a fever. Though the condition is a total misnomer, it is very real all the same. Watering, itching eyes, a constant sniffle, nasal stuffiness, postnasal drip, sneezing at the most inappropriate times, all must be endured by the hay fever sufferer during the various pollinating seasons of the plant world, depending on whether the victim is allergic to trees, grass, or weeds. At best, hay fever is annoying, a plain nuisance and very effective at robbing one of the social graces. At worst, it can lead to asthma, which can be a debilitating and disabling disease and sometimes fatal.

Some unfortunate allergic individuals suffer these same symptoms of rhinitis at various times of the year independent of the pollen seasons, even all year round. The allergens responsible for such perennial rhinitis are ubiquitous substances such as house dust or molds. Perennial rhinitis is more difficult to diagnose and frequently more difficult to treat and control than its pollen-produced cousin. For instance, how does one divorce the housewife from house dust? Not easily, I am sure.

The following symptoms can indicate allergic reactions in the respiratory system:

Constant coughing

Croup

Nasal polyps (watery swellings on the nasal mucosa which can obstruct breathing)

Recurrent infections and colds

Serous otitis ("glue ear," an inflammation which can lead to impaired hearing)

Rhinitis (inflammation of the nasal mucosa)

Swelling of glottis (the sound-producing apparatus of the larynx) and laryngitis

Frequent nosebleeds

Asthma

The gastrointestinal system from its beginning at the mouth to its end at the anus can register a number of discomforts in response to allergens, mainly but not exclusively to those ingested. Allergists are often tempted to call allergy to food the "hidden" allergy, since it is difficult to comprehend and often very hard to track down. Most of us find it perplexing that perfectly good, nourishing foods could produce such disastrous results as the following:

1. Mouth

Swelling, itching, burning of lips, tongue, gums and/or pharynx

Chapped and inflamed lips

Canker sores

Bad breath and an unpleasant taste

Geographical tongue (a patchy tongue that vaguely resembles a map)

2. Throat

Mucus overproduction resulting in constant clearing and coughing

A sensation of a lump in the throat

A sensation of difficulty in swallowing

3. Stomach

Heartburn

Nausea and perhaps vomiting

Sourness

Bloating and belching

Spasms of the opening between the stomach and duodenum

4. Intestines

Acute or subacute pain

Diarrhea and/or constipation

Blood in stool

Mucous colitis

5. Rectal area

    Itching of anal area

    Rectal bleeding

    Tenesmus (a persistent feeling that the bowel needs emptying)

    Inflammation of rectum and anus

Gastrointestinal symptoms of allergy may be so mild as to be dismissed with impatience by relatives and friends and even on occasion by physicians. No doubt, some patients have been told that they were simply neurotic or hypochondrial when in actuality some item in the diet or, more rarely, some allergen inhaled was producing the problem. On the other hand, gastrointestinal allergy symptoms can be so horrendous as to send the frightened patient hurrying to a physician pursued by fears of some dread disease. Naturally, the physician must rule out other potential problems before he or she can "think" allergy, and, as a matter of fact, other more grim possibilities do come first to mind. Gastrointestinal allergy can almost always be managed, a word employed more frequently in the treatment of allergy then the word cured, for although the symptoms of hypersensitivity may vanish, the condition itself usually persists. It could be said to be lying dormant, waiting to be reactivated by an allergen that slips by the barriers of self-control or vigilance.

The genito-urinary system is not immune either to the effects of the allergen-antibody battle. The allergic individual could suffer the following consequences of ingesting or even of inhaling an allergen:

The need to urinate frequently

Painful urination

Enuresis (incontinence, bed wetting; the child who has such difficulties should be assessed with allergy in mind as well as other possibilities)

Vaginal itching

The presence of significant serum protein in the urine after a period of standing

As if all of the above long list of symptoms were not enough, there are the autoimmune diseases in which muscles, bone, and the circulatory system can register hypersensitivity. Reactions in bone and muscle may result in pain and tenderness and rheumatoid arthritis, whereas blood vessel involvement may result in anemia, a too-ready bleeding of the mouth or skin on slight injury, a marked decrease in white blood corpuscles, and/or a disease called granulocytosis with symptoms of a high fever, weakness, and ulcers of the mouth, vagina, and rectum. We will delve further into the autoimmune diseases, the diseases against "self," in a later chapter.

Perhaps strangest of all are allergic reactions in the nervous system, for brain and nerve cells are not immune from an excessive clash of antibody and allergen. Although what actually takes place is still something of a mystery, it is believed that the vascular changes which occur in other body systems during an allergic reaction and which lead to edema and constriction also occur in the nervous system to produce a variety of symptoms ranging from headache to peculiar behavior. Some researchers believe that what happens is akin to the production of hives in the skin, especially when it occurs in the cranial area. Others suggest that the release of serotonin as well as of histamine that occurs during an allergic reaction plays a significant role. Serotonin, while stored in the main in the gastrointestinal system, also occurs in some quantity in the central nervous system. Originally, I was a skeptic about such reactions, but in my years of clinical practice, I have found many patients whose headaches and other nervous system disturbances disappeared when certain allergenic foods were eliminated from their diets. But to be quite honest about it, there is a great deal that we don't know about such reactions.

Finally, there is one serious consequence of being severely allergic, especially to insect venom or to drugs such as aspirin or penicillin or even to potent food allergens such as shellfish. This condition, anaphylaxis, can intensify so rapidly from initial symptoms to potentially fatal shock with falling blood pressure and respiratory difficulties that there is often little time to seek medical aid. Such a life-threatening reaction may begin mildly enough with itching around the eyes, widespread hives, a cough, and a vague feeling of anxiety and discomfort. In rapid succession, often within minutes of exposure to the allergen, the patient may complain of a constricted feeling in the chest, of dizziness and abdominal pain. He or she may begin to wheeze, be nauseated, vomit. Weakness, hoarseness of speech, confusion, and a terrible sensation of impending disaster may follow. The victim may become cyanotic as blood pressure falls steeply. Unconsciousness, coma, and death can follow.

All this can occur as the result of a single sting by a bee, a very small injection of penicillin, the ingestion of just a little of a potently allergenic food. Fortunately, it does not occur frequently, and it can be controlled and/or aborted, as I take great pains to demonstrate later in this book.

By now, the reader must be aware that allergy can wreak a good deal of havoc. We have touched on some of the factors which play a role in this odd clash of allergen and antibody, but our consideration has been brief. In the next chapter we explore at greater depth the things other than allergens which determine whether a hypersensitive individual will react to his or her nemesis at one time and not at another, whether an infection gives rise to allergy, and who among us are the allergic.

GLOSSARY

Intradermal: beneath the outer layer of the skin.

RAST: radioallergosorbent test.

Allergic march: progression of allergy diseases from colic to eczema to asthma.

Urticaria: hives.

Angioedema: giant hives; wheals accompanied by subcutaneous swelling or swelling of submucous tissues.

Nasal polyps: watery swellings or tumors.

Geographical tongue: patchy, denuded areas of the tongue.

Mucous colitis: inflammation of the colon accompanied by the production of a great deal of mucus.

SUMMARY

1. Although allergic reactions can occur in almost every body system, the skin, respiratory, and gastrointestinal systems are most frequently affected.

2. Steps in diagnosing allergy disease:

    Patient's history

    Physical examination

Laboratory tests

Skin tests and/or RAST

Elimination diet for food allergy

Patch tests for contact dermatitis

3. Anaphylactic shock reaction can be swift, severe, and sometimes fatal.

three

Allergy does not usually operate as a "lone wolf" disease. Although an allergen-antibody clash is the primary mechanism of an allergic reaction, whether or not that clash takes place at a given time under a given exposure to allergens in the environment may depend on other factors. There are times when the hypersensitive individual is more susceptible to that exposure and times when he or she is less vulnerable and may remain symptom free. This is truly a loaded gun cocked and ready to be fired, and although some severely allergic individuals need only an allergen alone to trigger the gun, many may not go off unless other factors are also at work.

Although they are not the "cause" of an allergic reaction, these triggers or factors can precipitate or aggravate symptoms of allergy disease. Dr. William C. Deamer has illustrated this phenomenon with a very lethal-looking weapon, which I reproduce on the next page with his kind permission.

For a more peaceful approach, let us observe the artwork of Dr. Frederick Speer, who illustrates this interplay of primary and secondary factors.

The Loaded Gun

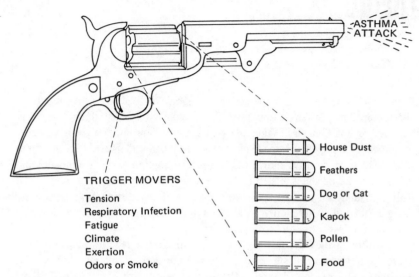

Causes of asthma: assumed versus actual. From William C. Deamer, "Environmental Control," in *Allergy and Immunology in Childhood,* Frederic Speer and Robert J. Dockhorn, eds., Springfield, IL: Charles C. Thomas, 1973, p. 383. Reprinted with permission.

Not to be outdone, I shall somewhat facetiously illustrate this hypothesis that factors, which form what many allergists dub the "allergic load," influence the production of symptoms in a large number of hypersensitive individuals. The story goes as follows:

It is an early fall day, warm, bright and sunny: an ideal day for fishing. We have, in fact, two gentlemen out in their respective boats on a lake, trying very hard to bring in some large-mouth bass. Both of our fishermen are allergic to ragweed, and unfortunately for them, the mild breeze is carrying the unseen enemy in their direction.

Fisherman 1 has brought a lunch of yogurt, carrot sticks, and an apple, a lunch that most allergists would agree is thoroughly nonallergenic even though some people might call it something else. Whatever else it is, we can all agree that it is surely a healthy meal. In any case, Fisherman 1 eats, enjoys, and goes right on serenely fishing, catching the big ones with nary a sniffle or sneeze.

Fisherman 2, however, has just downed a largish lunch of two hard-boiled eggs, a peanut butter sandwich, and a big chocolate bar. In addition, he was up late the night before, unable to sleep because of his anxiety about his impending divorce; thus he was both worried and weary. But he has just had a nibble except. . . he is seized by a paroxysm of sneezing so violent that the boat rocks, and the fish gets away. He begins to sniffle, and suddenly he is wheezing—asthma has struck!

Returning to Dr. Deamer's loaded gun, we can consider that ragweed pollen is the bullet for both our fishermen, but since Fisherman 1 is only mildly allergic to ragweed and since exposure is light and no other factors are at work to lower his tolerance, he remains symptom free. But, alas, Fisherman 2

The allergic cycle. From *Allergy and Immunology in Childhood,* Frederic Speer and Robert J. Dockhorn, eds., Springfield, IL: Charles C. Thomas, 1973, p. 226. Reproduced with permission.

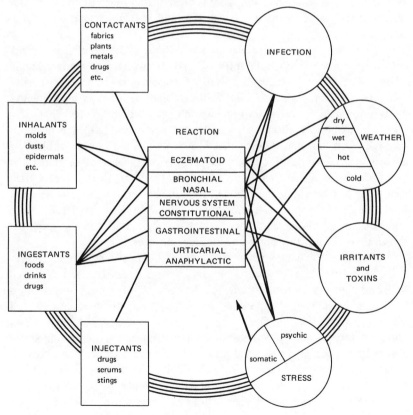

has a multitude of problems, beginning with the ragweed and doubling with the addition of eggs and chocolate, to both of which he is also sensitive. Then the additional factors of fatigue and emotional stress are enough to precipitate and aggravate his equally mild hypersensitivity to ragweed pollen and, literally, almost sink his boat. His tolerance level has been broached!

One of the most frequent questions patients ask me and one of the most difficult to answer is, why is my allergy suddenly worse at one time than another, or why did I develop allergy after all these years? I have found that the concept of the "allergic load," which I hasten to add is a hypothesis, not a scientific fact, is the most easily comprehended explanation. It is analogous to the often heard remark, "If I hadn't partied all night, I never would have caught this darn cold!" What is really being said is that the factors of loss of sleep, fatigue, and the unwise consumption of food and drink lowered resistance to the cold virus, and there is great truth in such a complaint. Our resistance to disease has its ups and downs, and so it is with our tolerance to allergens.

One factor suspected of playing a major role in determining an individual's tolerance level is another antibody, IgG. If IgE is the antibody villain in allergy, then IgG is probably the hero. We possess greater concentrations of IgG than other antibodies, which is fortunate since their conferring immunity on us is our main defense against disease. In relation to allergy, IgG appears to play a blocking role. Studies have indicated that when IgG concentrations rise, IgE levels fall. It is thought that IgG antibodies are capable of blocking allergen access to IgE antibodies, thus preventing the release of histamine that results from the allergen-antibody IgE clash. However, there is still a great deal to be learned about the action of IgG, and as of this writing we have not been able to establish a cause-and-effect relationship. High IgG levels do not always bring symptom relief for the hypersensitive, but recent research has shown that IgG probably plays a major blocking role.

Infection is a factor which has long been associated with allergy diseases, especially those of the respiratory system. Recent research has even indicated that viral infections enhance IgE-mediated histamine release; thus an allergic individual or one predisposed to allergy may be symptom free until suffering a viral infection. One study, not yet completed, of children with a family history of allergy demonstrated that half such children would suffer allergy before the age of five and that almost all such allergies were preceded by an upper respiratory infection, with a gap of about a month or less between the infection and the onslaught of allergy symptoms.

The role of infection in allergy diseases is very far from clear, however, for it is possible that the roles may be reversed on occasion, and the conditions allergy produces, especially in the respiratory system, may invite infective agents. An inflamed nasal mucosa, for instance, may serve as an open invitation to the cold virus. Thus the interrelationship of infection and allergy is still an ambiguous one, but that infection is an important factor is not in doubt. As we discuss the various allergy diseases later in this book, we examine that role in greater depth.

There is another factor that may have some influence in the production of allergy diseases, although the reader must understand that here I am theorizing to some extent. A lot has been said in recent years in and out of medical circles about the various influences of biological rhythms on living things. The circadian (daily) cycle has been of special interest and has been the most extensively studied. I am not speaking of horoscopes and the like, but rather of some sound scientific research on the physical and mental phases we pass through every 24 hours. In fact, all living things follow a recognizable pattern. We are all creatures of the day and night, the monthly phases of the moon, the recurring cycles of the seasons. We move through timeless fluctuations, which we do not yet thoroughly understand; yet we have just begun to realize that these forces affect us directly, mind and body.

In the circadian rhythm, which approximates the familiar 24-hour day, we alter a little with each passing hour and are not the same, say, at dawn as we are at dusk. For example, studies have shown that body temperature changes during this cycle peak in the afternoon or early evening for those of us we call the day hunters, peaking later in the evening for those who revel further into the night. Another study has demonstrated that poor sleepers arrive at rising time in the morning with below-normal body temperatures, while their opposites, those who sleep "like babies" and rise cheerfully with the alarm, generally exhibit "normal" temperatures. When the philosopher puts the end of a stick in the river, withdraws it, and puts it in again, he knows the river is not the same, that it has changed. And so it is with us from hour to hour, day to day, month to month, and year to year. In Nature nothing stands pat.

Some of the more pertinent studies for our subject of allergy are those delving into the effects of toxic substances during various periods of the circadian rhythm and those dealing with the varying potency of therapeutic drugs. As these studies have demonstrated, for instance, living things react differently to poisons at different times of the day, and a given dose will be more lethal at one time than at another. For example, an insecticide is lethal for about 10% of a given insect population at dawn, but if sprayed on the same species a few hours later, it will be fatal to some 90% of that population. Similarly, therapeutic drugs are more effective at optimum periods in the patient's daily cycle and markedly less effective at other periods. This, of course, is of vital interest to the medical profession. Drugs being administered on an arbitrary and rigid schedule, which does not coincide with the best of all times for the patient, may require heavier dosages to effect proper results, but this may increase the risk of side effects to accomplish what lesser dosages could do at the proper circadian moment. A case in point is chemotherapy for cancer victims. Healthy body cells have a daily cycle of mitosis (cell division), but cancer cells exhibit more random mitosis which may or may not synchronize with that of the healthy cells. Some chemotherapy drugs and radiation therapy halt cancer cell mitosis at any given time during the circadian cycle, but unless geared to healthy cell mitosis, they may also destroy healthy tissue cells. Thus if they are administered when healthy cells are not dividing, less benign tissue will be destroyed. Animal experiments have also demonstrated that certain kinds of tumor cells appear to be more highly susceptible to drugs at certain times during the daily rhythm than at others. This cycle of heightened susceptibility and of resistance also apparently varies from drug to drug; thus each drug's action appears to be more efficient at various stages of the cancer cell's cycle.

It is evident that there are great possibilities inherent in research into biological rhythms. Technically labeled *chronobiology,* this new knowledge may make it possible to prevent some health problems, and it is certain to help us to treat better many that do develop. It seems probable also that we may be able to predict the allergic individual's cycle of susceptibility so that he or she can avoid that which generates symptoms. Since avoidance is the keystone of control for much of allergy, this could be a major breakthrough.

Weather, too, can be a factor in allergy diseases, and it can be an especially significant factor in respiratory allergy, as might be expected. Asthma in particular seems to be aggravated by abrupt weather changes, by storm fronts, and by cold, windy days. It is apparently not so much the weather itself, although cold and heat and rain and dryness do play a role, but the abruptness of weather change that is the biggest factor. Sudden changes in barometric pressure, whether up or down, may affect the asthmatic, for instance, and cold, windy air may bring on nasal obstruction and rhinitis as well. Falling humidity may also be a factor, drying out nasal membranes to cause itching, irritation, and blockage. As we discuss in the chapter on asthma, the asthmatic individual can have some real difficulties with the weather.

Not to wander off on tangents, but to consider all interesting if not particularly scientific possibilities, let us consider that adjunct of weather, atmospheric ionization. Ions are charged atmospheric particles which are unstable, possessing either more or fewer electrons. Those possessing more are negative ions, those possessing fewer are positive. Ions are created when oxygen atoms are struck by cosmic rays, by light particles, or by other molecules. In the earth itself they are formed by radioactive bombardment. It is possible that all living things benefit by their presence, for studies have indicated that mice kept in an ion-free environment are twice as susceptible to a virus than control mice kept in a regular environment. Plants kept in an ion-free atmosphere demonstrate growth retardation. Because ions are quickly destroyed in the air when they collide with other particles, pollution may play a large part in de-ionizing the atmosphere, with all that that might mean for human health.

It has been demonstrated that positive ions have a direct effect on us, for when positive ionization is high, nasal mucous membranes dry; the nose and eyes itch and burn; the nose becomes obstructed; the throat is raw and dry. Breathing difficulties may result. Other physical changes include increased blood pressure, metabolism, and respiration.

Negative ions, on the other hand, have been shown to alleviate these symptoms and to promote a sense of well-being and health. Asthma and hay fever patients treated with negative-ion exposure reported improvement in their symptoms, but such improvement was short lived, and symptoms returned with a return to a normal environment.

It is of interest to note that negative ionization is supposed to be greater at higher altitudes and that positive ionization is more intense before the approach of thunderstorms.

And as a definite aside, ionization apparently also affects our emotional set as well. Under the influence of positive ions, serotonin release is increased. A hormone, it affects the nervous system, constricts blood vessels, and slows the healing process of wounds and lesion. An increase in serotonin can cause feelings of irritability and belligerence and increased sensitivity to pain.

A good example of positive ionization of the atmosphere occurs when the fohn wind blows, such as the Santa Ana wind of California. The fohn is hot and dry and occurs when a strong wind blows over the mountains and is dragged downward on the lee side. When it blows, people are apt to become tense, angry, or depressed. Swiss studies have demonstrated an increase in suicides and admissions to mental institutions when the fohn occurs there, and in Israel, where it is called the sharav, it is claimed that some young people become violent while older people slip into states of depression.

Back to allergy. We have now indicated that allergic individuals are like loaded guns, primed to fire, and that they are literally surrounded by various factors which can trigger and/or aggravate their problems.

Who are these "loaded guns"?

A good many of them are children. Approximately one in four or one in five children in this country is allergic to something. A number of studies and surveys suggest that around 80% of allergy diseases begin during the first 14 years of life. One study concluded that about 95% of these allergic youngsters developed symptoms of allergy before they were four years old. Such figures demonstrate the need for early recognition and treatment of allergy diseases, for the allergic child may become the chronically ill and very allergic adult. Not only that, but like many other chronic diseases, allergy can trail a number of physical and emotional problems in its wake, as we discuss in a later chapter. It is better to "head 'em off at the pass" than risk the allergic march to asthma and other complications.

It appears that the percentage of allergy disease in relation to other chronic diseases does not change much during the years 0 to 16, for allergy remains somewhere in the neighborhood of 34% of the chronic diseases suffered by children during this period. Thus approximately one-third of American children suffering from chronic ill health are suffering from allergy diseases. Such statistics underline the importance of allergy training for pediatricians and general practitioners.

It is also significant that more boys develop allergy than do girls, although exactly why remains something of a mystery. Some studies indicate that boys suffer especially from asthma and eczema, in fact, almost twice as often as do girls, with the ratio even greater in some regions of the country.

A good deal of research has gone into an attempt to identify factors that initiate allergy in predisposed children with an eye, of course, to preventing sensitization when and where possible. Respiratory infections, as we noted earlier, appear to play a significant role in the development of asthma; thus the more such infections can be avoided, the less the chance of subsequent asthma. Some studies have pointed an accusing finger at early surgery, especially surgery on children under two years of age, as being a factor in the later development of allergy, especially of rhinitis and asthma. In one study of 115 children who had undergone surgery for pyloric stenosis, a condition in infancy of an excessively narrow opening between the stomach and the duodenum, resulting in frequent and explosive vomiting, some 18% subsequently developed asthma and 23% developed hay fever, percentages which were markedly higher than would be expected in that particular population at large. Another study of boys who had been operated on to repair hernias during the first year of life revealed an even higher rate of subsequent allergy. Asthma was reported in 34% of the youngsters and hay fever in 21%. This compares to a random sample of children with no history of early surgery whose incidence of asthma was 4.4% and of hay fever was 9.8%. The authors of these and other studies have suggested that if surgery is elective and can be postponed until after the age of two, there might be a corresponding reduction of major respiratory allergies.

The great difficulty in doing scientific studies is that frequently there is someone waiting in the wings to bring out results of *their* study to flatly contradict yours. In this case, there are other studies that have found no significant increase in allergy subsequent to early surgery. In a survey conducted among mothers of children operated on for pyloric stenosis in the first year of life, the results were that of 294 interviewed, 45 reported that their children had later developed respiratory allergy. This amounted to 15%, with 2.3% of these children developing asthma. A national survey has indicated that between 10 to 20% of American youngsters suffer respiratory allergies in the population at large, with 3% of these exhibiting symptoms of asthma. Thus the authors of the above study concluded that surgery before two years of age had no real impact on the later development of respiratory allergies.

And that, like many another pressing question in the literature of allergy, is where we stand at the moment. What we do know is that in one form or another allergy does loom large in childhood health problems and, perhaps, on some childhood behavior problems as well. This latter possibility is explored in a later chapter.

Allergy tends to make its first appearance before the age of four, frequently in infancy with symptoms of colic and/or eczema. There is a popular notion among some physicians and many parents that children will "outgrow" their allergies, but the fact is that they often simply exchange one allergy for another. A child may begin with symptoms of gastrointestinal allergy to milk. Later he or she may react to pollen or house dust or animal dander with respiratory allergy symptoms.

Since allergy can become chronic and since chronic disease can become debilitating as well as something of a handicap, especially for the young, we should realize that untreated and uncontrolled allergy can cause a youngster a good deal of discomfort and emotional stress. Growing up is difficult enough to cope with as it is, without additional problems of chronic ill health. Lasting stigmata of severe allergy can range from mouthbreathing, with possible orthodontic abnormalities, to personality and behavior problems.

Adults may also suffer chronic allergy diseases, for we have just begun to recognize that there is a growing segment of the population whose allergies relate to occupation. Workers in cotton mills may become sensitized to cotton dusts and suffer a debilitating and disabling lung disease called bisinosis. Workers in granaries may have problems with smut and rust spores which are released in quantity from the grains they handle. Bakers may become allergic to flour to develop baker's asthma. Even housewives are not immune to occupational allergy, for they can become hypersensitive to the house dust mite which resides in uncountable numbers under our roofs. As we go on to examine the various allergy diseases and the allergens which cause them, we will explore further various occupational hypersensitivities.

By this time, the reader should be aware that those among us who are genetically predisposed to allergy are truly "loaded guns." Whether the gun fires or not may depend, in part at least, on these other factors we have discussed. Or it may not. A great deal depends on the tolerance of the individual and the extent and duration of exposure to an allergen. A great deal depends, too, on the potency of the allergen, so let us next take a good look at allergens—what they are, where found, and when.

GLOSSARY

Circadian cycle: the daily biological rhythm.

Pyloric stenosis: an excessively narrow opening between the stomach and duodenum.

SUMMARY

1. Allergens are the primary cause of allergy diseases.
2. A number of secondary factors play a role in precipitating and/or aggravating allergy disease.
3. Immunoglobulin G (IgG) is suspected of being a blocking antibody capable of interfering with the allergen-antibody clash.

4. Infection is one of the most important factors in respiratory allergy diseases.

5. Biological rhythms may influence allergy disease to some extent.

6. Weather and sudden changes in weather can be a significant factor in allergy, respiratory allergy especially.

PART II

ALLERGENS— WHERE AND WHEN

four

To the misfortune of hypersensitive individuals, many seed-bearing plants, the Spermatophyta, conduct their sex life at considerable distance, depending on the wind to ensure the propagation of their species. Woe to the allergy predisposed who happen to get in the way! Such unwitting interference is still called rose or hay fever, although roses and hay as such usually have little or nothing to do with the disastrous results, nor does such an allergy often sport a fever. Actually, the misnomer rose fever arose from the fact that symptoms of rhinitis caused by pollinating plants frequently occurred while roses were in full bloom. For much the same reason, the term hay fever stuck because people noticed that they sniffled and sneezed when in proximity of the grasses and weeds of hay fields. Another mistaken belief is that goldenrod is a prime offender, since it is often turning the landscape yellow while ragweed is casting its potent pollen abroad.

Generally, it isn't the plants that display bright and perfumed flowers that affect the allergic. Such plants depend mainly on the insect world to help them spread their species, for they have discovered the secret of enticement.

Of Plants and Pollen

With nectar and color and sweet smells, they attract bees and other insects, even birds on occasion and, once in a while, bats, all of whom fly off to visit other flowers with pollen grains sticking to their hairs or feathers. Pollen, which is analogous to sperm in animals, is caught by the sticky part of the female element of the visited plant, the carpel, then transmitted to the ovary section where the seeds are formed.

To complete this brief elementary biology lesson, let us note that when a plant possesses both male and female elements, it is termed monoecious. When it possesses only one or the other, it is called dioecious. Pollen is produced and held in readiness in the anthers, tiny podlike formations on the ends of the stamens. When the petals of the flower open in the morning, the plant is in business. The anthers will split a little, and pollen will emerge. The mysterious thing in all this is, how are the pollens of foreign species rejected when they are transported by wing or wind? How does the flower know which pollen belongs to its own species? We don't really know, but it is speculated that there is some mechanism for recognition of self, perhaps in the form of chemical receptors.

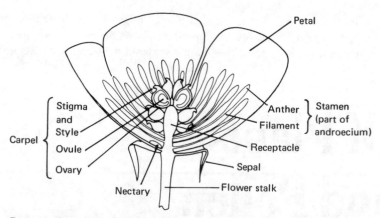

Cross-section view of a self-pollinating flower.

In any case, the beautiful and the fragrant, the insect pollinated, called the entomophilous, are not the chief villains in allergy. Although it is infrequent, it can happen, however, and perhaps the most bizarre of insect pollenosis (allergy due to plants that are insect pollinated) has occurred among a few health-food fans who have taken to eating bee pollen, which has been highly touted for its health-giving properties. One lumberjack who consumed a tablespoon of the stuff ended up in the hospital emergency room with anaphylactic shock symptoms. A woman who consumed no more than a teaspoon and a half developed airway obstruction and breathing difficulties within 45 minutes of downing her bee pollen. An analysis of some bee pollens sold in health-food stores revealed the presence of dandelion pollen grains, and since dandelion is a member of the same plant family, Compositae, as ragweed, it is possible that some people allergic to ragweed can cross-react to dandelion. This may explain why the woman in the case above reacted, although she may have been allergic to bee venom. In the cases of three other individuals who suffered severe anaphylactic shock reactions after eating bee pollen containing dandelion pollen, ragweed allergies were mild. Investigators suggest that the difference between the mild reactions to inhaled pollen in contrast to the life-threatening reactions to ingested pollen could lie in the degree of exposure, since the bee pollen possibly contained billions of pollen grains to the tablespoon. Sunflowers also belong to the same plant family as ragweed, and similar severe allergic reactions to the ingestion of sunflower seeds have been reported.

When it comes to the main offenders in inhaled pollenosis, we must turn to the not-so-showy-world of grasses, trees, and weeds, the anemophilous

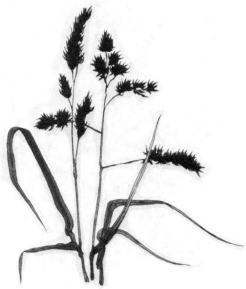

Orchard grass (*Dactylis glomerata*), also known as cocksfoot, dew, or hard grass, favors moisture and partial shade throughout temperate North America. It sheds its pollen in May and June.

Drawings on pp. 41–46 are reproduced with permission from Fisons Corporation.

or wind-pollinated plants. Because the breezes they must depend on to propagate their kind are apt to be chancy, they literally fill the air with tons of pollen, much of it protein in nature. One statistic guaranteed to frighten the hay-fever sufferer is that a single ragweed plant can produce some 2 trillion pollen grains during its lifespan. Someone with a mathematical turn of mind has calculated that one acre of ragweed can produce 60 pounds of pollen during its pollinating, late-summer season. It would be a chore to sack the stuff, if you could see it, that is, to cart it away; yet the wind may carry it for many miles. When abundant, it can sometimes be seen as yellowish clouds in the sky on warm, dry days with a stiff prevailing breeze. When the wind dies and/or humidity rises, pollen fallout may occur to form yellowish mats in lakes and streams. Alaskan pollen has been found in Oregon, and rural New York State pollen has found its way to Wall Street. Fortunately, however, much of this astonishing production moves only a few feet from the parent plant.

Those plants which are especially spiteful in producing pollenosis in

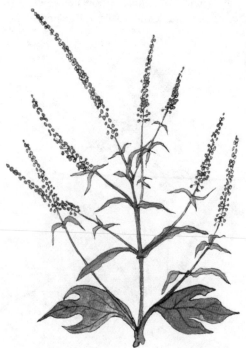

Giant ragweed (*Ambrosia trifida*), whose seed is carried great distances by streams and rivers and whose abundant pollen is windblown from August to September, ranges in distribution from Quebec to North Carolina and west to Colorado.

humans follow a set of conditions called Thommen's postulates. The plants must be widely distributed, be extravagant in their production of pollen, produce airborne pollen that is allergenic in nature, and bear seeds.

In addition to the plants themselves, a number of other factors affect the amount of pollen in the air. Although light summer showers have little effect on pollination in progress, heavy rains tend to prevent distribution and help destroy the pollen more quickly. Since most pollen is released in the early morning hours, usually between 6 and 9 A.M., the damage is done before those summer thunderstorms so frequent in the late afternoon appear over the horizon to damp things down. High humidity, however, does tend to weight pollen down and to restrict its movement. Hot, dry, sunny days, on the other hand, lighten pollen so that the slightest breeze can waft it far and wide.

Seashores can be a refuge for hay-fever victims, since winds are generally from offshore, but as they blow inland, they are unmerciful for the landlubbers some distance from the sea. Ragweed sufferers are apt to rejoice when the first heavy frost appears, but unfortunately their jubilation is pre-

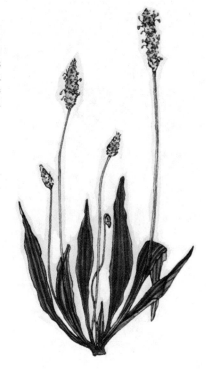

English plantain (*Plantago lanceolata*), also known as ribgrass, can be found throughout the United States and Canada. With help from the wind, this species is the only one to shed enough pollen and is abundant enough to cause allergy, beginning to flower in April and peaking in May and June.

mature, for most of the pollen has been produced and can be cast still upon the wind. Allergic individuals residing in mild climates find no real end to the hay-fever season, since grass and weed pollens are about almost the year-round.

Of all the pollen-producing plants in the United States ragweed is the chief villain and the main cause for hay fever and other allergy problems. Unhappily, it is truly abundant across the land except on the extreme west coast and Alaska. The misery this feathery plant causes is so extensive that efforts have been made in some areas to get rid of it, but, unfortunately, ragweed has discovered the secret of survival. Its seeds are capable of germinating years after they have been sown, and wherever man turns the earth with plow or bulldozer, he is actually helping ragweed to flourish. If it is any consolation, ragweed roots help prevent erosion, since they grow deep and since ragweed thrives on poor soil.

The nature of pollen itself is as important as is its mode and efficiency

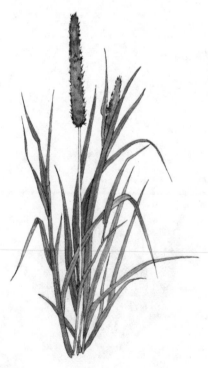

Timothy (*Phleum pratense*) flowers in June and July, sheds enormous quantities of pollen, and is one of the worst causes of allergy symptoms in early summer. It is found in fields and waste places throughout the United States.

of transport. Various studies have fractionated pollen in an attempt to sepa-rate out its various components, especially those that are allergenic. Grass pollen, for instance, was found to have at least 15 allergens and at least three have been discovered in ragweed pollen.

The size of pollen grains is also important when it comes to their ability to inflict misery. Those grains that are very small can pass beyond the guardian structures of the nose into the smaller ducts of the bronchi, where they can inflict mild to severe health problems, depending on the allergenic nature of the pollen and the degree of hypersensitivity of the individual they invade. Heavier pollen, such as is produced by large, bright flowers, never really gets off the ground. To be airborne, pollen is somewhere between 15 to 50 microns in diameter (a micron is one millionth of a meter; about 1/25,000 part of an inch), small enough to be invasive of the human nasal structures. Somewhere in the neighborhood of 100 plant species produce pollen that can be significantly responsible for human (and animal) allergy diseases.

Red oak (*Quercus rubra*) is the best known and common name for a group of North American trees. Oak pollen causes more allergy than most trees. Pollen grains are gen-erally shed in May, but this can vary depending upon the climatic factors of the locality.

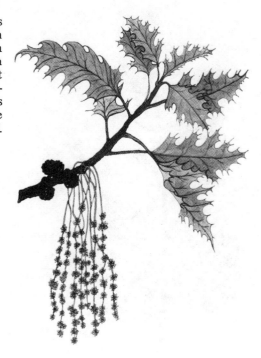

The mechanism by which pollen causes hay fever and other allergies is still somewhat mysterious. Research has indicated a number of possibilities. Lysozyme (the stuff of our tears, saliva, and nasal mucus) is an enzyme with antibacterial properties. It is known to be capable of dissolving the exterior coating of pollen grains, thus releasing the allergenic protein substances within. These, it is believed, are absorbed by the nasal mucosa to come in contact with sensitized mast cells in the submucosa with a resulting antibody response of edema and infiltration of eosinophil cells, whose action, alas, is not thoroughly understood. As we noted in Chapter 2, their increased presence is often indicative of allergy. One theory of their role postulates that they assist in the repair of damaged mast cells. In any case, the allergic reaction to allergenic pollen is immediate, and the greater the exposure and the longer its duration, the worse the resulting obstruction.

A knowledge of what plants are pollinating and when in any given area is essential for the physician and for the patient who suffers from hay fever or other allergy symptoms to pollen, for avoidance is the keystone for such

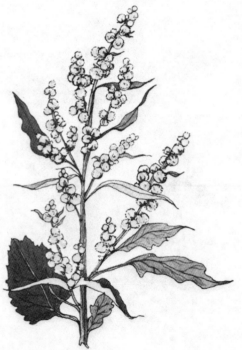

Lambs quarters (*Chenopodium album*) is a tall, succulent herb found throughout North America. From August until frost these plants are wind pollinated. Although they do not shed excessive amounts of pollen, their abundance can be an important cause of allergy symptoms.

MAJOR BOTANICAL AREAS

The United States and Canada are divided into twenty-one (21) regions. The regions are generally composed of contiguous areas having similar climatic and geographical features. State and Province boundaries may be used for easy identification whenever possible, but other boundaries may be identified by counties within states, or major geographical features.

Region I

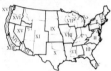

North Atlantic U.S.A.

STATES:

Connecticut	Maine
Massachusetts	New Hampshire
New Jersey	New York
Pennsylvania	Rhode Island
Vermont	

VEGETATION:

Trees—Appalachian oak forest and northern hardwood forest (beech, birch, hemlock, and maple).

Grasses—Several genera, naturalized and/or cultivated for hay and lawns, although inconspicuous, are very abundant and significant in hayfever.

Weeds—Although relatively few species of weeds are important, their widespread abundance and heavy pollination over a long season make them important hayfever plants.

INDEX TREES: (Pollinating Season—Late Winter through Spring)

BOX ELDER/MAPLE (*Acer spp.*)
BIRCH (*Betula spp.*)
OAK (*Quercus spp.*)
HICKORY (*Carya ovata*)
ASH (*Fraxinus americana*)
PINE (*Pinus strobus*)
SYCAMORE (*Platanus occidentalis*)
COTTONWOOD/POPLAR (*Populus deltoides*)
ELM (*Ulmus americana*)

INDEX GRASSES: (Pollinating Season—Spring through Early Summer)

REDTOP (*Agrostis alba*)
ORCHARD (*Dactylis glomerata*)
FESCUE (*Festuca elatior*)
TIMOTHY (*Phleum pratense*)
BLUEGRASS/JUNEGRASS (*Poa spp.*)

INDEX WEEDS: (Pollinating Season—Summer through Early Fall)

LAMB'S QUARTERS (*Chenopodium album*)
RAGWEED, GIANT & SHORT (*Ambrosia spp.*)
COCKLEBUR (*Xanthium strumarium*)
PLANTAIN (*Plantago lanceolata*)
DOCK/SORREL (*Rumex spp.*)

Region II

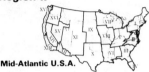

Mid-Atlantic U.S.A.

STATES:

Delaware	District of Columbia
Maryland	North Carolina
Virginia	

VEGETATION:

Trees—Appalachian oak forest and oak-hickory-pine forest.

Grasses—Several genera, naturalized and/or cultivated for hay and lawns, although inconspicuous, are very abundant and significant in hayfever.

Weeds—Although relatively few species of weeds are important, their widespread abundance and heavy pollination over a long season make them important hayfever plants.

INDEX TREES: (Pollinating Season—Late Winter through Spring)

BOX ELDER/MAPLE (*Acer spp.*)
BIRCH (*Betula nigra*)
CEDAR/JUNIPER (*Juniperus virginiana*)
OAK (*Quercus spp.*)
HICKORY/PECAN (*Carya spp.*)
WALNUT (*Juglans nigra*)
MULBERRY (*Morus spp.*)
ASH (*Fraxinus americana*)
COTTONWOOD/POPLAR (*Populus deltoides*)
HACKBERRY (*Celtis occidentalis*)
ELM (*Ulmus americana*)

INDEX GRASSES: (Pollinating Season—Spring through Early Summer)

REDTOP (*Agrostis alba*)
VERNALGRASS (*Anthoxanthum sp.*)
BERMUDAGRASS (*Cynodon dactylon*)
ORCHARDGRASS (*Dactylis glomerata*)
RYEGRASS (*Elymus & lolium spp.*)
TIMOTHY (*Phleum pratense*)
BLUEGRASS/JUNEGRASS (*Poa spp.*)
JOHNSONGRASS (*Sorghum halepense*)

INDEX WEEDS: (Pollinating Season—Summer through Early Fall)

PIGWEED (*Amaranthus retroflexus*)
LAMB'S QUARTERS (*Chenopodium album*)
MEXICAN FIREBUSH (*Kochia scoparia*)
RAGWEED, GIANT & SHORT (*Ambrosia spp.*)
COCKLEBUR (*Xanthium strumarium*)
PLANTAIN (*Plantago lanceolata*)
DOCK/SORREL (*Rumex spp.*)

From *Pollen Guide for Allergy* with permission from Hollister Stier.

Region III

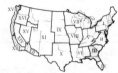

South Atlantic U.S.A.

STATES:
Florida, Northern, (above Orlando)
Georgia   South Carolina

VEGETATION:
Trees — Oak-hickory-pine forest and southern mixed forest (beech, oak, pine).

Grasses — Several genera, naturalized and/or cultivated for hay and lawns, although inconspicuous, are very abundant and significant in hayfever.

Weeds — Although relatively few species of weeds are important, their widespread abundance and heavy pollination over a long season make them important hayfever plants.

INDEX TREES: (Pollinating Season — Late Winter through Spring)
BOX ELDER/MAPLE (*Acer spp.*)
BIRCH (*Betula nigra*)
CEDAR/JUNIPER (*Juniperus virginiana*)
OAK (*Quercus spp.*)
HICKORY/PECAN (*Carya spp.*)
WALNUT (*Juglans nigra*)
MESQUITE (*Prosopis juliflora*)
MULBERRY (*Morus spp.*)
ASH (*Fraxinus americana*)
COTTONWOOD/POPLAR (*Populus deltoides*)
HACKBERRY (*Celtis occidentalis*)
ELM (*Ulmus americana*)

INDEX GRASSES: (Pollinating Season — Spring through Early Summer)
REDTOP (*Agrostis alba*)
VERNALGRASS (*Anthoxanthum sp.*)
BERMUDAGRASS (*Cynodon dactylon*)
ORCHARDGRASS (*Dactylis glomerata*)
RYEGRASS (*Elymus & Lolium spp.*)
FESCUE (*Festuca elatior*)
TIMOTHY (*Phleum pratense*)
BLUEGRASS/JUNEGRASS (*Poa spp.*)
JOHNSONGRASS (*Sorghum halepense*)

INDEX WEEDS: (Pollinating Season — Summer through Early Fall)
LAMB'S QUARTERS (*Chenopodium album*)
RAGWEED, GIANT & SHORT (*Ambrosia spp.*)
SAGEBRUSH (*Artemisia spp.*)
COCKLEBUR (*Xanthium strumarium*)
PLANTAIN (*Plantago lanceolata*)
DOCK/SORREL (*Rumex spp.*)

Region IV

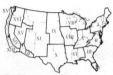

Subtropic Florida

STATES:
Florida, Southern (Below Orlando)

VEGETATION:
Trees — Southern mixed forest, palmetto prairie, and everglades.

Grasses — Several genera, naturalized and/or cultivated for hay and lawns, although inconspicuous, are very abundant and significant in hayfever.

Weeds — Although relatively few species of weeds are important, their widespread abundance and heavy pollination over a long season make them important hayfever plants.

INDEX TREES: (Pollinating Season — Winter through Spring)
BOX ELDER (*Acer negundo*)
CEDAR/JUNIPER (*Juniperus virginiana*)
OAK (*Quercus spp.*)
PECAN (*Carya pecan*)
PRIVET (*Ligustrum lucidum*)
PALM (*Cocos plumosa*)
AUSTRALIAN PINE (BEEFWOOD) (*Casuarina equisetifolia*)
SYCAMORE (*Platanus occidentalis*)
COTTONWOOD/POPLAR (*Populus deltoides*)
ELM (*Ulmus americana*)
BRAZILIAN PEPPERTREE (FLORIDA HOLLY) (*Schinus terebinthifolius*)
BAYBERRY (WAX MYRTLE) (*Myrica spp.*)
MELALEUCA (*Melaleuca sp.*)

INDEX GRASSES: (Pollinating Season — Spring through Early Summer)
REDTOP (*Agrostis alba*)
BERMUDAGRASS (*Cynodon dactylon*)
SALTGRASS (*Distichlis sp.*)
BAHIAGRASS (*Paspalum notatum*)
CANARYGRASS (*Phalaris minor*)
BLUEGRASS/JUNEGRASS (*Poa spp.*)
JOHNSONGRASS (*Sorghum halepense*)

INDEX WEEDS: (Pollinating Season — Summer through Early Fall)
PIGWEED (*Amaranthus spinosus*)
LAMB'S QUARTERS (*Chenopodium album*)
RAGWEED, GIANT & SHORT (*Ambrosia spp.*)
SAGEBRUSH (*Artemisia spp.*)
MARSH ELDER/POVERTY WEED (*Iva spp.*)
DOCK/SORREL (*Rumex spp.*)
PLANTAIN (*Plantago lanceolata*)

Region V

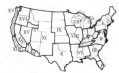

The Greater Ohio Valley

STATES:

Indiana	Kentucky
Ohio	Tennessee
West Virginia	

VEGETATION:

Trees—Mixed forest (beech, maple, oak), beech-maple forest, and oak-hickory forest.

Grasses—Several genera, naturalized and/or cultivated for hay and lawns, although inconspicuous, are very abundant and significant in hayfever.

Weeds—Although relatively few species of weeds are important, their widespread abundance and heavy pollination over a long season make them important hayfever plants.

INDEX TREES: (Pollinating Season—Late Winter through Spring)
BOX ELDER/MAPLE (*Acer spp.*)
BIRCH (*Betula nigra*)
OAK (*Quercus rubra*)
HICKORY (*Carya ovata*)
WALNUT (*Juglans nigra*)
ASH (*Fraxinus americana*)
SYCAMORE (*Platanus occidentalis*)
COTTONWOOD/POPLAR (*Populus deltoides*)
ELM (*Ulmus americana*)

INDEX GRASSES: (Pollinating Season—Spring through Early Summer)
REDTOP (*Agrostis alba*)
BERMUDAGRASS (*Cynodon dactylon*)
ORCHARDGRASS (*Dactylis glomerata*)
FESCUE (*Festuca elatior*)
RYEGRASS (*Lolium spp.*)
TIMOTHY (*Phleum pratense*)
BLUEGRASS/JUNEGRASS (*Poa spp.*)
JOHNSONGRASS (*Sorghum halepense*)

INDEX WEEDS: (Pollinating Season—Summer through Early Fall)
WATERHEMP (*Acnida tamariscina*)
PIGWEED (*Amaranthus retroflexus*)
LAMB'S QUARTERS (*Chenopodium album*)
RAGWEED, GIANT & SHORT (*Ambrosia spp.*)
SAGEBRUSH (*Artemisia spp.*)
COCKLEBUR (*Xanthium strumarium*)
DOCK/SORREL (*Rumex spp.*)
PLANTAIN (*Plantago lanceolata*)

Region VI

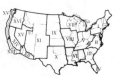

South Central U.S.A.

STATES:

Alabama	Arkansas
Louisiana	Mississippi

VEGETATION:

Trees—Southern flood plain forest, surrounded by oak-hickory-pine forest and oak-hickory forest.

Grasses—Several genera, naturalized and/or cultivated for hay and lawns, although inconspicuous, are very abundant and significant in hayfever.

Weeds—Although relatively few species of weeds are important, their widespread abundance and heavy pollination over a long season make them important hayfever plants.

INDEX TREES: (Pollinating Season—Late Winter through Spring)
BOX ELDER/MAPLE (*Acer spp.*)
CEDAR/JUNIPER (*Juniperus virginiana*)
OAK (*Quercus spp.*)
HICKORY/PECAN (*Carya spp.*)
WALNUT (*Juglans nigra*)
ASH (*Fraxinus americana*)
SYCAMORE (*Platanus occidentalis*)
COTTONWOOD/POPLAR (*Populus deltoides*)
HACKBERRY (*Celtis occidentalis*)
ELM (*Ulmus americana*)

INDEX GRASSES: (Pollinating Season—Spring through Early Summer)
REDTOP (*Agrostis alba*)
BERMUDAGRASS (*Cynodon dactylon*)
ORCHARDGRASS (*Dactylis glomerata*)
RYEGRASS (*Lolium spp.*)
TIMOTHY (*Phleum pratense*)
BLUEGRASS/JUNEGRASS (*Poa spp.*)
JOHNSONGRASS (*Sorghum halepense*)

INDEX WEEDS: (Pollinating Season—Summer through Early Fall)
CARELESSWEED/PIGWEED (*Amaranthus spp.*)
LAMB'S QUARTERS (*Chenopodium album*)
RAGWEED, GIANT & SHORT (*Ambrosia spp.*)
SAGEBRUSH (*Artemisia spp.*)
MARSH ELDER/POVERTY WEED (*Iva spp.*)
COCKLEBUR (*Xanthium strumarium*)
PLANTAIN (*Plantago lanceolata*)
DOCK/SORREL (*Rumex spp.*)

Region VII

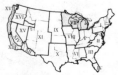

The Northern Midwest

STATES:
Michigan   Minnesota
Wisconsin

VEGETATION:

Trees—Northern hardwood and Great Lakes pine forests, bluestem prairie and oak savannahs.

Grasses—Several genera, naturalized and/or cultivated for hay and lawns, although inconspicuous, are very abundant and significant in hayfever.

Weeds—Although relatively few species of weeds are important, their widespread abundance and heavy pollination over a long season make them important hayfever plants.

INDEX TREES: (Pollinating Season—Late Winter through Spring)

BOX ELDER/MAPLE (*Acer spp.*)
ALDER (*Alnus incana*)
BIRCH (*Betula spp.*)
OAK (*Quercus rubra*)
HICKORY (*Carya ovata*)
WALNUT (*Juglans nigra*)
ASH (*Fraxinus americana*)
SYCAMORE (*Platanus occidentalis*)
COTTONWOOD/POPLAR (*Populus deltoides*)
ELM (*Ulmus americana*)

INDEX GRASSES: (Pollinating Season—Spring through Early Summer)

REDTOP (*Agrostis alba*)
BROME (*Bromus inermis*)
ORCHARDGRASS (*Dactylis glomerata*)
FESCUE (*Festuca elatior*)
RYEGRASS (*Lolium spp.*)
CANARYGRASS (*Phalaris arundinacea*)
TIMOTHY (*Phleum pratense*)
BLUEGRASS/JUNEGRASS (*Poa spp.*)

INDEX WEEDS: (Pollinating Season—Summer through Early Fall)

WATERHEMP (*Acnida tamariscina*)
LAMB'S QUARTERS (*Chenopodium album*)
RUSSIAN THISTLE (*Salsola kali*)
RAGWEED, GIANT & SHORT (*Ambrosia spp.*)
MARSH ELDER/POVERTY WEED (*Iva spp.*)
COCKLEBUR (*Xanthium strumarium*)
DOCK/SORREL (*Rumex spp.*)
PIGWEED (*Amaranthus retroflexus*)
PLANTAIN (*Plantago lanceolata*)

Region VIII

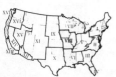

The Central Midwest

STATES:
Illinois   Iowa
Missouri

VEGETATION:

Trees—Mixed bluestem prairie and oak-hickory forest, and relatively large mixed areas.

Grasses—Several genera, naturalized and/or cultivated for hay and lawns, although inconspicuous, are very abundant and significant in hayfever.

Weeds—Although relatively few species of weeds are important, their widespread abundance and heavy pollination over a long season make them important hayfever plants.

INDEX TREES: (Pollinating Season—Late Winter through Spring)

BOX ELDER/MAPLE (*Acer spp.*)
BIRCH (*Betula nigra*)
OAK (*Quercus spp.*)
HICKORY (*Carya ovata*)
WALNUT (*Juglans nigra*)
MULBERRY (*Morus spp.*)
ASH (*Fraxinus americana*)
SYCAMORE (*Platanus occidentalis*)
COTTONWOOD/POPLAR (*Populus deltoides*)
ELM (*Ulmus americana*)

INDEX GRASSES: (Pollinating Season—Spring through Early Summer)

REDTOP (*Agrostis alba*)
BERMUDAGRASS (*Cynodon dactylon*)
ORCHARDGRASS (*Dactylis glomerata*)
RYEGRASS (*Lolium spp.*)
TIMOTHY (*Phleum pratense*)
BLUEGRASS/JUNEGRASS (*Poa spp.*)
JOHNSONGRASS (*Sorghum halepense*)
CORN (*Zea mays*)

INDEX WEEDS: (Pollinating Season—Summer through Early Fall)

PIGWEED (*Amaranthus retroflexus*)
LAMB'S QUARTERS (*Chenopodium album*)
MEXICAN FIREBUSH (*Kochia scoparia*)
RUSSIAN THISTLE (*Salsola kali*)
RAGWEED, GIANT, SHORT & WESTERN (*Ambrosia spp.*)
MARSH ELDER/POVERTY WEED (*Iva spp.*)
PLANTAIN (*Plantago lanceolata*)
DOCK/SORREL (*Rumex spp.*)
WATERHEMP (*Acnida tamariscina*)

Region IX

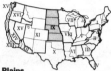

The Great Plains

STATES:

Kansas	Nebraska
North Dakota	South Dakota

VEGETATION:

Trees—Mixed prairies; predominant trees cultivated.

Grasses—This region is predominantly grassland, but the more important hayfever grasses are cultivated for hay or lawns, or are naturalized pests.

Weeds—Although relatively few species of weeds are important, their widespread abundance and heavy pollination over a long season make them important hayfever plants.

INDEX TREES: (Pollinating Season—Late Winter through Spring)
BOX ELDER/MAPLE (*Acer spp.*)
ALDER (*Alnus incana*)
BIRCH (*Betula spp.*)
HAZELNUT (*Corylus americana*)
OAK (*Quercus macrocarpa*)
HICKORY (*Carya ovata*)
WALNUT (*Juglans nigra*)
ASH (*Fraxinus americana*)
COTTONWOOD/POPLAR (*Populus deltoides*)
ELM (*Ulmus americana*)

INDEX GRASSES: (Pollinating Season—Spring through Early Summer)
QUACKGRASS/WHEATGRASS (*Agropyron spp.*)
REDTOP (*Agrostis alba*)
BROME (*Bromus inermis*)
ORCHARDGRASS (*Dactylis glomerata*)
RYEGRASS (*Elymus & Lolium spp.*)
FESCUE (*Festuca elatior*)
TIMOTHY (*Phleum pratense*)
BLUEGRASS/JUNEGRASS (*Poa spp.*)

INDEX WEEDS: (Pollinating Season—Summer through Early Fall)
WATERHEMP (*Acnida tamariscina*)
PIGWEED (*Amaranthus retroflexus*)
LAMB'S QUARTERS (*Chenopodium album*)
MEXICAN FIREBUSH (*Kochia scoparia*)
RUSSIAN THISTLE (*Salsola kali*)
RAGWEED, FALSE, GIANT, SHORT &
    WESTERN (*Ambrosia spp.*)
SAGEBRUSH (*Artemisia spp.*)
MARSH ELDER/POVERTY WEED (*Iva spp.*)
COCKLEBUR (*Xanthium strumarium*)
PLANTAIN (*Plantago lanceolata*)
DOCK/SORREL (*Rumex spp.*)

Region X

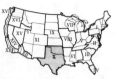

Southwestern Grasslands

STATES:

Oklahoma	Texas

VEGETATION:

Trees—Shrub savannah in the west and south, central and northern mixed prairies, and eastern oak-hickory-pine forests.

Grasses—This region is predominantly grassland, but the more important hayfever grasses are cultivated for hay or lawns, or are naturalized pests.

Weeds—Although relatively few species of weeds are important, their widespread abundance and heavy pollination over a long season make them important hayfever plants.

INDEX TREES: (Pollinating Season—Late Winter through Spring)
BOX ELDER (*Acer negundo*)
CEDAR/JUNIPER (*Juniperus virginiana*)
OAK (*Quercus virginiana*)
MESQUITE (*Prosopis juliflora*)
MULBERRY (*Morus spp.*)
ASH (*Fraxinus americana*)
COTTONWOOD/POPLAR (*Populus deltoides*)
ELM (*Ulmus americana*)

INDEX GRASSES: (Pollinating Season—Spring through Early Summer)
QUACKGRASS/WHEATGRASS (*Agropyron spp.*)
REDTOP (*Agrostis alba*)
BERMUDAGRASS (*Cynodon dactylon*)
ORCHARDGRASS (*Dactylis glomerata*)
FESCUE (*Festuca elatior*)
RYEGRASS (*Lolium spp.*)
TIMOTHY (*Phleum pratense*)
BLUEGRASS/JUNEGRASS (*Poa spp.*)
JOHNSONGRASS (*Sorghum halepense*)

INDEX WEEDS: (Pollinating Season—Summer through Early Fall)
WATERHEMP (*Acnida tamariscina*)
CARELESS WEED/PIGWEED (*Amaranthus spp.*)
SALTBUSH/SCALE (*Atriplex spp.*)
LAMB'S QUARTERS (*Chenopodium album*)
MEXICAN FIREBUSH (*Kochia scoparia*)
RUSSIAN THISTLE (*Salsola kali*)
RAGWEED, FALSE, GIANT, SHORT &
    WESTERN (*Ambrosia spp.*)
SAGEBRUSH (*Artemisia spp.*)
MARSH ELDER/POVERTY WEED (*Iva spp.*)
COCKELBUR (*Xanthium strumarium*)
DOCK/SORREL (*Rumex spp.*)
PLANTAIN (*Plantago lanceolata*)

Region XI

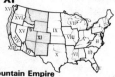

Rocky Mountain Empire

STATES:

Arizona (Mountainous)   Colorado
Idaho (Mountainous)   Montana
New Mexico   Utah
Wyoming

VEGETATION:

Trees — Mixed prairies and steppes to pinyon-juniper woodlands and mixed conifer forests, from lower elevation and latitude to higher.

Grasses — Several genera, naturalized and/or cultivated for hay and lawns, although inconspicuous, are very abundant and significant in hay-fever.

Weeds — Although relatively few species of weeds are important, their widespread abundance and heavy pollination over a long season make them important hayfever plants.

INDEX TREES: (Pollinating Season — Late Winter through Spring)
BOX ELDER (*Acer negundo*)
ALDER (*Alnus incana*)
BIRCH (*Betula fontinalis*)
CEDAR/JUNIPER (*Juniperus scopulorum*)
OAK (*Quercus gambelii*)
ASH (*Fraxinus americana*)
PINE (*Pinus spp.*)
COTTONWOOD/POPLAR (*Populus deltoides*) (*sargentii*)
ELM (*Ulmus spp.*)

INDEX GRASSES: (Pollinating Season — Spring through Early Summer)
QUACKGRASS/WHEATGRASS (*Agropyron spp.*)
REDTOP (*Agrostis alba*)
BROME (*Bromus inermis*)
BERMUDAGRASS (*Cynodon dactylon*)
ORCHARDGRASS (*Dactylis glomerata*)
RYEGRASS (*Elymus & Lolium spp.*)
FESCUE (*Festuca elatior*)
TIMOTHY (*Phleum pratense*)
BLUEGRASS/JUNEGRASS (*Poa spp.*)

INDEX WEEDS: (Pollinating Season — Summer through Early Fall)
WATERHEMP (*Acnida tamariscina*)
PIGWEED (*Amaranthus retroflexus*)
SALTBUSH/SCALE (*Atriplex spp.*)
SUGARBEET (*Beta vulgaris*)
LAMB'S QUARTERS (*Chenopodium album*)
MEXICAN FIREBUSH (*Kochia scoparia*)
RUSSIAN THISTLE (*Salsola kali*)
RAGWEED, FALSE, GIANT, SHORT & WESTERN (*Ambrosia spp.*)
SAGEBRUSH (*Artemisia spp.*)
MARSH ELDER/POVERTY WEED (*Iva spp.*)
COCKLEBUR (*Xanthium strumarium*)
PLANTAIN (*Plantago lanceolata*)
DOCK/SORREL (*Rumex spp.*)

Region XII

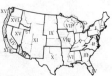

The Arid Southwest

STATES:
Arizona   Southern California (S.E. Desert)

VEGETATION:

Trees — Creosote bush shrub and palo verde-cactus shrub; predominant trees cultivated.

Grasses — Several genera, naturalized and/or cultivated for hay and lawns wherever possible, although inconspicuous, are significant in hayfever.

Weeds — Although relatively few species of weeds are important, their widespread abundance and heavy pollination over a long season make them important hayfever plants. Many of these are shrubby relatives of weeds common to regions with more precipitation.

INDEX TREES: (Pollinating Season — Winter through Spring)
CYPRESS (*Cupressus arizonica*)
CEDAR/JUNIPER (*Juniperus californica*)
MESQUITE (*Prosopis juliflora*)
ASH (*Fraxinus velutina*)
OLIVE (*Olea europaea*)
COTTONWOOD/POPLAR (*Populus fremontii*)
ELM (*Ulmus parvifolia*)

INDEX GRASSES: (Pollinating Season — Spring through Early Summer)
BROME (*Bromus spp.*)
BERMUDAGRASS (*Cynodon dactylon*)
SALTGRASS (*Distichlis sp.*)
RYEGRASS (*Elymus & Lolium spp.*)
CANARYGRASS (*Phalaris minor*)
BLUEGRASS/JUNEGRASS (*Poa spp.*)

INDEX WEEDS: (Pollinating Season — Summer through Early Fall)
CARELESS WEED (*Amaranthus palmeri*)
IODINE BUSH (*Allenrolfea occidentalis*)
SALTBUSH/SCALE (*Atriplex spp.*)
LAMB'S QUARTERS (*Chenopodium album*)
RUSSIAN THISTLE (*Salsola kali*)
ALKALI-BLITE (*Suaeda sp.*)
RAGWEED, FALSE, SLENDER & WESTERN (*Ambrosia spp.*)
SAGEBRUSH (*Artemisia spp.*)
SILVER RAGWEED (*Dicoria canescens*)
BURRO BRUSH (*Hymenoclea salsola*)

Region XIII

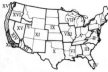

Southern Coastal California

STATES:
California, Southern Coastal

VEGETATION:

Trees—Chaparral and coastal sagebrush shrub to California steppe; many species of ornamental trees cultivated.

Grasses—Several genera, naturalized and/or cultivated for hay and lawns, although inconspicuous, are very abundant and significant in hayfever.

Weeds—Although relatively few species of weeds are important, their widespread abundance and heavy pollination over a long season make them important hayfever plants.

INDEX TREES: (Pollinating Season—Late Winter through Spring)
BOX ELDER (*Acer negundo*)
CYPRESS (*Cupressus arizonica*)
OAK (*Quercus agrifolia*)
WALNUT (*Juglans spp.*)
ACACIA (*Acacia spp.*)
MULBERRY (*Morus spp.*)
EUCALYPTUS (*Eucalyptus sp.*)
ASH (*Fraxinus velutina*)
OLIVE (*Olea europaea*)
SYCAMORE (*Platanus racemosa*)
COTTONWOOD/POPLAR (*Populus trichocarpa*)
ELM (*Ulmus spp.*)

INDEX GRASSES: (Pollinating Season—Spring through Early Summer)
OATS (*Avena spp.*)
BROME (*Bromus spp.*)
BERMUDAGRASS (*Cynodon dactylon*)
ORCHARDGRASS (*Dactylis glomerata*)
SALTGRASS (*Distichlis sp.*)
RYEGRASS (*Elymus & Lolium spp.*)
FESCUE (*Festuca elatior*)
BLUEGRASS/JUNEGRASS (*Poa spp.*)
JOHNSONGRASS (*Sorghum halepense*)

INDEX WEEDS: (Pollinating Season—Summer through Early Fall)
CARELESSWEED/PIGWEED (*Amaranthus spp.*)
SALTBUSH/SCALE (*Atriplex spp.*)
LAMB'S QUARTERS (*Chenopodium album*)
RUSSIAN THISTLE (*Salsola kali*)
RAGWEED, FALSE, SLENDER & WESTERN (*Ambrosia spp.*)
SAGEBRUSH (*Artemisia spp.*)
COCKLEBUR (*Xanthium strumarium*)
PLANTAIN (*Plantago lanceolata*)
DOCK/SORREL (*Rumex spp.*)

Region XIV

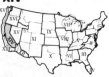

The Central California Valley

STATES:
California (Sacramento and San Joaquin Valleys)

VEGETATION:

Trees—California steppe bordered by California oakwoods; many species of ornamental, nut, and fruit trees cultivated.

Grasses—Several genera, naturalized and/or cultivated for hay and lawns, although inconspicuous, are very abundant and significant in hayfever.

Weeds—Although relatively few species of weeds are important, their widespread abundance and heavy pollination over a long season make them important hayfever plants.

INDEX TREES: (Pollinating Season—Late Winter through Spring)
BOX ELDER (*Acer negundo*)
ALDER (*Alnus rhombifolia*)
BIRCH (*Betula fontinalis*)
CYPRESS (*Cupressus arizonica*)
OAK (*Quercus lobata*)
PECAN (*Carya pecan*)
WALNUT (*Juglans spp.*)
ASH (*Fraxinus velutina*)
OLIVE (*Olea europaea*)
SYCAMORE (*Platanus acerifolia*)
COTTONWOOD/POPLAR (*Populus fremontii*)
ELM (*Ulmus spp.*)

INDEX GRASSES: (Pollinating Season—Spring through Early Summer)
REDTOP (*Agrostis alba*)
OATS (*Avena spp.*)
BROME (*Bromus spp.*)
BERMUDAGRASS (*Cynodon dactylon*)
ORCHARDGRASS (*Dactylis glomerata*)
SALTGRASS (*Distichlis sp.*)
RYEGRASS (*Elymus & Lolium spp.*)
FESCUE (*Festuca elatior*)
CANARYGRASS (*Phalaris minor*)
TIMOTHY (*Phleum pratense*)
BLUEGRASS/JUNEGRASS (*Poa spp.*)
JOHNSONGRASS (*Sorghum halepense*)

INDEX WEEDS: (Pollinating Season—Summer through Early Fall)
PIGWEED (*Amaranthus retroflexus*)
SALTBUSH/SCALE (*Atriplex spp.*)
SUGARBEET (*Beta vulgaris*)
LAMB'S QUARTERS (*Chenopodium album*)
RUSSIAN THISTLE (*Salsola kali*)
RAGWEED, FALSE, SLENDER & WESTERN (*Ambrosia spp.*)
SAGEBRUSH (*Artemisia spp.*)
COCKLEBUR (*Xanthium strumarium*)
PLANTAIN (*Plantago laceolata*)
DOCK/SORREL (*Rumex spp.*)

Region XV

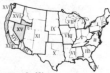

The Intermountain West

STATES:
Idaho (Southern)   Nevada

VEGETATION:

Trees — Sagebrush steppe, saltbush-greasewood and Great Basin sagebrush shrub; predominant trees cultivated.

Grasses — Several genera, naturalized and/or cultivated for hay and lawns wherever possible, although inconspicuous, are significant in hayfever.

Weeds — Although relatively few species of weeds are important, their widespread abundance and heavy pollination over a long season make them important hayfever plants. Many of these are shrubby relatives of weeds common to regions with more precipitation.

INDEX TREES: (Pollinating Season — Late Winter through Spring)
BOX ELDER (*Acer negundo*)
ALDER (*Alnus incana*)
BIRCH (*Betula fontinalis*)
CEDAR/JUNIPER (*Juniperus utahensis*)
ASH (*Fraxinus americana*)
SYCAMORE (*Platanus occidentalis*)
COTTONWOOD/POPLAR (*Populus trichocarpa*)
ELM (*Ulmus spp.*)

INDEX GRASSES: (Pollinating Season — Spring through Early Summer)
QUACKGRASS/WHEATGRASS (*Agropyron spp.*)
REDTOP (*Agrostis alba*)
BROME (*Bromus inermis*)
BERMUDAGRASS (*Cynodon dactylon*)
ORCHARDGRASS (*Dactylis glomerata*)
SALTGRASS (*Distichlis sp.*)
RYEGRASS (*Elymus & Lolium spp.*)
FESCUE (*Festuca elatior*)
TIMOTHY (*Phleum pratense*)
BLUEGRASS/JUNEGRASS (*Poa spp.*)

INDEX WEEDS: (Pollinating Season — Summer through Early Fall)
PIGWEED (*Amaranthus retroflexus*)
IODINE BUSH (*Allenrolfea occidentalis*)
SALTBUSH/SCALE (*Atriplex spp.*)
LAMB'S QUARTERS (*Chenopodium album*)
MEXICAN FIREBUSH (*Kochia scoparia*)
RUSSIAN THISTLE (*Salsola kali*)
RAGWEED, FALSE, SLENDER &
  WESTERN (*Ambrosia spp.*)
SAGEBRUSH (*Artemisia spp.*)
MARSH ELDER/POVERTY WEED (*Iva spp.*)
COCKLEBUR (*Xanthium strumarium*)
PLANTAIN (*Plantago lanceolata*)
DOCK/SORREL (*Rumex spp.*)

Region XVI

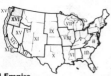

The Inland Empire

STATES:
Oregon (Central and Eastern)
Washington (Central and Eastern)

VEGETATION:

Trees — Bluegrass-fescue-wheatgrass grasslands and sagebrush steppe bordered by coniferous forests; predominant trees cultivated.

Grasses — This region is predominantly grassland, but the more important hayfever grasses are cultivated for seed, hay, or lawns, or are naturalized pests.

Weeds — Although relatively few species of weeds are important, their widespread abundance and heavy pollination over a long season make them important hayfever plants.

INDEX TREES: (Pollinating Season — Late Winter through Spring)
BOX ELDER (*Acer negundo*)
ALDER (*Alnus incana*)
BIRCH (*Betula fontinalis*)
OAK (*Quercus garryana*)
WALNUT (*Juglans nigra*)
PINE (*Pinus spp.*)
COTTONWOOD/POPLAR (*Populus trichocarpa*)
WILLOW (*Salix lasiandra*)

INDEX GRASSES: (Pollinating Seaspn — Spring through Early Summer)
QUACKGRASS/WHEATGRASS (*Agropyron spp.*)
REDTOP (*Agrostis alba*)
VERNALGRASS (*Anthoxanthum sp.*)
BROME (*Bromus inermis*)
ORCHARDGRASS (*Dactylis glomerata*)
RYEGRASS (*Elymus & Lolium spp.*)
VELVETGRASS (*Holcus lanatus*)
TIMOTHY (*Phleum pratense*)
BLUEGRASS/JUNEGRASS (*Poa spp.*)

INDEX WEEDS: (Pollinating Season — Summer through Early Fall)
PIGWEED (*Amaranthus retroflexus*)
SALTBUSH/SCALE (*Atriplex spp.*)
LAMB'S QUARTERS (*Chenopodium album*)
MEXICAN FIREBUSH (*Kochia scoparia*)
RUSSIAN THISTLE (*Salsola kali*)
RAGWEED, FALSE, GIANT, SHORT &
  WESTERN (*Ambrosia spp.*)
SAGEBRUSH (*Artemisia spp.*)
MARSH ELDER/POVERTY WEED (*Iva spp.*)
PLANTAIN (*Plantago lanceolata*)
DOCK/SORREL (*Rumex spp.*)

Region XVII

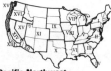

Cascade Pacific Northwest

STATES:

California (Northwestern)   Oregon (Western)
Washington (Western)

VEGETATION:

Trees — Mixed coniferous forests; hardwoods primarily cultivated.

Grasses — Several genera, naturalized and/or cultivated for hay and lawns, although inconspicuous, are very abundant and significant in hayfever. Grass seed is produced extensively in parts of this region.

Weeds — Although relatively few species of weeds are important, their widespread abundance and heavy pollination over a long season make them important hayfever plants.

INDEX TREES: (Pollinating Season — Late Winter through Spring)
BOX ELDER (*Acer negundo*)
ALDER (*Alnus rhombifolia*)
BIRCH (*Betula fontinalis*)
HAZELNUT (*Corylus cornuta*)
OAK (*Quercus garryana*)
WALNUT (*Juglans regia*)
ASH (*Fraxinus oregona*)
COTTONWOOD/POPLAR (*Populus trichocarpa*)
WILLOW (*Salix lasiandra*)
ELM (*Ulmus pumila*)

INDEX GRASSES: (Pollinating Season — Spring through Early Summer)
BENTGRASS (*Agrostis maritima*)
VERNALGRASS (*Anthoxanthum sp.*)
OATS (*Avena spp.*)
BROME (*Bromus inermis*)
BERMUDAGRASS (*Cynodon dactylon*)
ORCHARDGRASS (*Dactylis glomerata*)
SALTGRASS (*Distichlis sp.*)
RYEGRASS (*Elymus & Lolium spp.*)
FESCUE (*Festuca elatior*)
VELVETGRASS (*Holcus lanatus*)
CANARYGRASS (*Phalaris arundinacea*)
TIMOTHY (*Phleum pratense*)
BLUEGRASS/JUNEGRASS (*Poa spp.*)

INDEX WEEDS: (Pollinating Season — Summer through Early Fall)
PIGWEED (*Amaranthus retroflexus*)
SALTBUSH/SCALE (*Atriplex spp.*)
LAMB'S QUARTERS (*Chenopodium album*)
RUSSIAN THISTLE (*Salsola kali*)
RAGWEED, FALSE, GIANT, SHORT & WESTERN (*Ambrosia spp.*)
SAGEBRUSH (*Artemisia spp.*)
COCKELBUR (*Xanthium strumarium*)
PLANTAIN (*Plantago lanceolata*)
DOCK/SORREL (*Rumex spp.*)

Region C-I

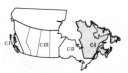

Atlantic Provinces & Quebec

PROVINCES:

Prince Edward Island   Nova Scotia
New Brunswick   Newfoundland
Quebec

VEGETATION:

Trees — From south to north, mixed wood forests and boreal forests open into woodlands and tundras through Quebec and Newfoundland, Acadian forests in the other Provinces.

Grasses — Several genera, naturalized and/or cultivated for hay and lawns, are very abundant and more significant than the native grasses in hayfever.

Weeds — Although relatively few species of weeds are important, their abundance in agricultural and urban areas makes them important hayfever plants.

INDEX TREES: (Pollinating Season — Late Winter through Spring)
BOX ELDER (Manitoba Maple) (*Acer negundo*)
HARD MAPLE (Sugar) (*Acer saccharum*)
TAG ALDER (Speckled) (*Alnus incana*)
PAPER BIRCH (White) (*Betula papyrifera*)
BEECH (*Fagus grandifolia*)
WHITE ASH (*Fraxinus americana*)
GREEN ASH (*Fraxinus pennsylvanica*)
BUTTERNUT (*Juglans cinerea*)
SYCAMORE (*Platanus occidentalis*)
BALSAM POPLAR (*Populus balsamifera*)
TREMBLING ASPEN (*Populus tremuloides*)
BUR OAK (*Quercus macrocarpa*)
BLACK WILLOW (*Salix nigra*)
AMERICAN ELM (White) (*Ulmus americana*)

INDEX GRASSES: (Pollinating Season — Spring through Early Summer)
QUACKGRASS (Couch) (*Agropyron repens*)
REDTOP (*Agrostis alba*)
BROME (*Bromus sp.*)
ORCHARDGRASS (*Dactylis glomerata*)
RYEGRASS (*Elymus/Lolium spp.*)
TIMOTHY (*Phleum pratense*)
BLUEGRASS (*Poa spp.*)

INDEX WEEDS: (Pollinating Season — Summer through Early Fall)
REDROOT PIGWEED (*Amaranthus retroflexus*)
RAGWEED (*Ambrosia spp.*)
LAMB'S QUARTERS (*Chenopodium album*)
PLANTAIN (*Plantago lanceolata*)
DOCK/SORREL (*Rumex spp.*)
RUSSIAN THISTLE (*Salsola kali*)

Region C-II

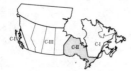

Ontario

PROVINCE:
Ontario

VEGETATION:

Trees—From south to north, mixed wood forests and boreal forests open into woodlands and tundras.

Grasses—Several genera, naturalized and/or cultivated for hay and lawns, are very abundant and more significant than the native grasses in hayfever.

Weeds—Although relatively few species of weeds are important, their abundance in agricultural and urban areas makes them important hayfever plants.

INDEX TREES: (Pollinating Season—Late Winter through Spring)
BOX ELDER (Manitoba Maple) (*Acer negundo*)
HARD MAPLE (Sugar) (*Acer saccharum*)
TAG ALDER (Speckled) (*Alnus incana*)
PAPER BIRCH (White) (*Betula papyrifera*)
BEECH (*Fagus grandifolia*)
WHITE ASH (*Fraxinus americana*)
GREEN ASH (*Fraxinus pennsylvanica*)
BUTTERNUT (*Juglans cinerea*)
SYCAMORE (*Platanus occidentalis*)
BALSAM POPLAR (*Populus balsamifera*)
ASPEN (*Populus tremuloides*)
BUR OAK (*Quercus macrocarpa*)
BLACK WILLOW (*Salix nigra*)
AMERICAN ELM (White) (*Ulmus americana*)
CHINESE ELM (Siberian) (*Ulmus pumila*)

INDEX GRASSES: (Pollinating Season—Spring through Early Summer)
QUACKGRASS (Couch) (*Agropyron repens*)
REDTOP (*Agrostis alba*)
BROME (*Bromus sp.*)
ORCHARDGRASS (*Dactylis glomerata*)
RYEGRASS (*Elymus/Lolium spp.*)
TIMOTHY (*Phleum pratense*)
BLUEGRASS (*Poa spp.*)

INDEX WEEDS: (Pollinating Season—Summer through Early Fall)
REDROOT PIGWEED (*Amaranthus retroflexus*)
RAGWEED (*Ambrosia spp.*)
LAMB'S QUARTERS (*Chenopodium album*)
ENGLISH PLANTAIN (*Plantago lanceolata*)
DOCK/SORREL (*Rumex spp.*)
RUSSIAN THISTLE (*Salsola kali*)

Region C-III

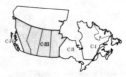

Prairie Provinces and Eastern British Columbia

PROVINCES:

Alberta	Eastern British Columbia
Manitoba	Saskatchewan

VEGETATION:

Trees—The southern third of the region is grassland and parkland, where the predominant trees are found only along watercourses or are cultivated. Cordilleran forests are in the west, mixed wood forests in the north, and boreal forests in the northern most parts.

Grasses—The more populous part of this region is predominately grassland, but the more important hayfever grasses are cultivated for hay or lawns, or are naturalized pests.

Weeds—Although relatively few species of weeds are important in Canada, there are several more species in this region; their abundance in agricultural and urban areas making them important hayfever plants.

INDEX TREES: (Pollinating Season—Late Winter through Spring)
BOX ELDER (Manitoba maple) (*Acer negundo*)
TAG ALDER (Speckled-Mountain) (*Alnus incana*)
PAPER BIRCH (White) (*Betula papyrifera*)
GREEN ASH (*Frexinus pennsylvanica*)
BALSAM POPLAR (*Populus balsamifera*)
TREMBLING ASPEN (*Populus tremuloides*)
BUR OAK (*Quercus macrocarpa*)
WILLOW (Yellow) (*Salix sp.*)
CHINESE ELM (Siberian) (*Ulmus pumila*)

INDEX GRASSES: (Pollinating Season—Spring through Early Summer)
QUACKGRASS (Couch) WHEATGRASS (*Agropyron spp.*)
REDTOP (*Agrostis alba*)
COMMON WILD OATS (*Avena fatua*)
BROME (*Bromus sp.*)
ORCHARD GRASS (*Dactylis glomerata*)
RYEGRASS (*Elymus/Lolium spp.*)
TIMOTHY (*Phleum pratense*)
BLUEGRASS (*Poa spp.*)

INDEX WEEDS: (Pollinating Season—Summer through Early Fall)
REDROOT PIGWEED (*Amaranthus retroflexus*)
RAGWEED (*Ambrosia spp.*)
LAMB'S QUARTERS (*Chenopodium album*)
SAGEBRUSH (*Artemisia spp.*)
MARSHELDER/POVERTY WEED (*Iva spp.*)
ENGLISH PLANTAIN (*Plantago lanceolata*)
DOCK/SORREL (*Rumex spp.*)
RUSSIAN THISTLE (*Salsola kali*)

Region C-IV

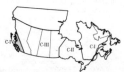

Western British Columbia & Vancouver Island
PROVINCES:
Western British Columbia   Vancouver Island

VEGETATION:

Trees—Except for the steppe, where the predominant trees are found only along watercourses or are cultivated, this region is cordilleran forest.

Grasses—Several genera, naturalized and/or cultivated for hay and lawns, are very abundant and more significant than the native grasses in hayfever.

Weeds—Although relatively few species of weeds are important, their abundance in agricultural and urban areas makes them important hayfever plants.

INDEX TREES: (Pollinating Season—Late Winter through Spring)
- BOX ELDER (Manitoba Maple) (*Acer negundo*)
- RED ALDER (*Alnus rubra*)
- SITKA ALDER (*Alnus sinuata*)
- PAPER BIRCH (White) (*Betula papyrifera*)
- SYCAMORE (*Platanus occidentalis*)
- BLACK COTTONWOOD (*Populus trichocarpa*)
- TREMBLING ASPEN (*Populus tremuloides*)
- DOUGLAS FIR (*Pseudotsuga menziesii*)
- GARRY'S OAK (*Quercus garryana*)
- YELLOW WILLOW (Pacific) (*Salix lasiandra*)
- CHINESE ELM (Siberian) (*Ulmus pumila*)

INDEX GRASSES: (Pollinating Season—Spring through Early Summer)
- QUACKGRASS (Couch) (*Agropyron repens*)
- REDTOP (*Agrostis alba*)
- TALL OAT GRASS (*Arrhenatherum elatius*)
- COMMON WILD OATS (*Avena fatua*)
- BROME (*Bromus sp.*)
- ORCHARDGRASS (*Dactylis glomerata*)
- RYEGRASS (*Elymus/Lolium spp.*)
- TIMOTHY (*Phleum pratense*)
- BLUEGRASS (*Poa spp.*)

INDEX WEEDS: (Pollinating Season—Summer through Early Fall)
- REDROOT PIGWEED (*Amaranthus retroflexus*)
- RAGWEED (*Ambrosia spp.*)
- LAMB'S QUARTERS (*Chenopodium album*)
- MARSHELDER/POVERTY WEED (*Iva spp.*)
- ENGLISH PLANTAIN (*Plantago lanceolata*)
- DOCK/SORREL (*Rumex spp.*)
- RUSSIAN THISTLE (*Salsola kali*)

Region: Alaska
Alaska
STATE:
Alaska

VEGETATION:

Typical hayfever species of the three plant forms, viz. trees, grasses, and weeds, are found in the southern coastal region which forms an arc from the southeasternmost point of the state northward, westward, then southward to the Alaska Peninsula. As a whole, the state has three principal vegetation types:

1. Dense sitka spruce and western hemlock forests. These trees are generally considered of very minor significance in allergy, if significant at all. However, alder, aspen, birch, and willow may be found in clearings and near watercourses, and may be associated with grasses and some weeds in the early stages of plant succession.

2. Less dense forests of birches and white spruce. The birches may be the most significant hayfever trees because they form such extensive forests.

3. Tundra and tundra-like, characterized by low vegetation, in the Aleutian Islands, the Bering Sea Coast and the Arctic Slope. Very cold winters and very cool moist summers are detrimental to tree growth. Grasses are predominant, but (as in tropical regions) the humidity and precipitation are so great that whatever airborne pollen is shed is not likely to remain airborne very long.

Index grasses and weeds are most common in the temperate agricultural and urban regions. The whole hayfever season is short, from three to six months according to latitude, elevation, and proximity to the seacoasts.

INDEX TREES: (Pollinating Season—Spring)
- ALDER (*Alnus incana*)
- ASPEN (*Populus tremuloides*)
- BIRCH (*Betula papyrifera*)
- CEDAR (*Thuja plicata*)
- HEMLOCK (*Tsuga hetrophylla*)
- PINE (*Pinus contorta*)
- POPLAR (*Populus balsamifera*)
- SPRUCE (*Picea sitchensis*)
- WILLOW (*Salix spp.*)

INDEX GRASSES: (Pollinating Season—Late Spring-Summer)
- BLUEGRASS/JUNEGRASS (*Poa spp.*)
- BROME (*Bromus inermis*)
- CANARYGRASS (*Phalaris arundinacea*)
- FESCUE (*Festuca rubra*)
- ORCHARDGRASS (*Dactylis glomerata*)
- QUACKGRASS/WHEATGRASS (*Agropyron spp.*)
- REDTOP (*Agrostis alba*)
- RYEGRASS (*Lolium perenne*)
- TIMOTHY (*Phleum pratense*)

INDEX WEEDS: (Pollinating Season—Summer)
- BULRUSH (*Scirpus sp.*)
- DOCK/SORREL (*Rumex spp.*)
- LAMB'S QUARTERS (*Chenopodium album*)
- NETTLE (*Urtica dioica*)
- PLANTAIN (*Plantago lanceolata*)
- SAGEBRUSH/WORMWOOD (*Artemisa spp.*)
- SEDGE (*Carex spp.*)
- SPEARSCALE (*Atriplex patula*)

inhalant problems. Tree pollens, for instance, generally start the pollen season in much of the country, beginning in March and running through mid-June. Grass pollens arrive on the scene generally in May and remain through July. Weeds come in various seasons, but ragweed pollen abounds from mid-August through September. These seasons vary a little, of course, depending on the region of the country.

In recent years weather reports in some areas of the country have listed pollen counts. How they arrive at such counts is interesting, varying as it does for different pollens and for different conditions. Gravitational methods have been used for many years, and one such method (the Durham sampler) is so simple that a physician or allergic patient could build one (or have it built) and be able to make an office-roof or window-ledge count with relatively good results. Two horizontal metal plates are separated by 3-inch supports. The slide holder is set in the middle and about 1 inch above the bottom plate. Glass microslides coated with soft glycerin jelly are set in place and left for 24 hours. The slides are then removed, and a 22-millimeter-square cover slip is set over the slide as a counting field, and the whole examined under a microscope. (The allergic patient curious enough to keep track of pollen may have to go forth for the above item.) The pollen is tallied as so much per square centimeter of slide surface.

More accurate volumetric techniques, including suction devices and rotating arm impactors, are employed for more precise readings, especially in research projects. Whatever the method, pollen counts as announced in the media should be taken with a grain of salt, for any given individual's exposure could be quite different, depending on when and where the count was taken in relation to the individual. It should also be remembered that the accuracy has its limitations; thus there is no need to get excited if the pollen count sounds high.

Pollen is pervasive in its season, but it is also a part of the natural world and has been present in the human environment from the beginning. In the next chapter we tackle a totally different kind of plant which, although it does not produce pollen, can cause a great deal of allergy. So let us move on to the fungi, those strange chlorophyll-less members of the plant world, and to mites, an equally strange insect member of the order Acarina.

GLOSSARY

Spermatophyta: seed-bearing plants.

Stamen: male sex organ of plant with filament bearing the anther, which contains the pollen.

Carpel: female sex organ of plant with ovary at base and sticky (usually) stigma at top.

Monoecious: plants which possess both male and female elements.

Dioecious: plants which possess only male or only female elements.

Entomophilous: insect-pollinated plants.

Anemophilous: wind-pollinated plants.

SUMMARY

1. Not all pollen-producing plants cause allergies.

2. Light, small pollens, highly allergenic in nature, are the chief offenders in allergy diseases.

3. About 100 species of plants produce offending pollens.

4. A number of factors influence the pollination of anemophilous plants: weather (rain or sunshine), wind, humidity, and general climate.

5. Thommen's postulates for a hay fever plant are:

   It must be a spermatophyte.

   It must have wide distribution.

   It must produce abundant pollen.

   Its pollen must be light.

   Its pollen must be allergenic.

6. Trees, grasses, and weeds pollinate in different seasons which vary somewhat in different regions of North America.

7. Pollen counts as reported in the media may have limited relevance for the allergy sufferer and limited accuracy.

five

I have lumped molds and mites together, not only because they are alliterate but because they are ubiquitous and highly successful plants and animals. Both are found just about everywhere on earth, except, perhaps, on the ice-caps at the Poles, and I am not sure that, if the hunt were on, they wouldn't be found up and down there.

I admit that I did choose the word *mold* for the alliteration of this chapter's title, but what I am really going to discuss are the fungi, of which molds are a part. The fungi are that part of the plant world that cannot synthesize food from water and carbon dioxide with the help of the sun, for they contain no chlorophyll. Thus they are preordained to a parasitic existence or to obtain their sustenance from decaying matter. In the first role they can cause a number of diseases for humans, ranging from ringworm and athletes foot to hypersensitivity pneumenitis, a serious lung condition. In the latter role they hasten the processes of disintegration. It has been said that without the fungi whole forests would disappear under the accumulations of their own dead leaves. When such processes of decay form our rich soil we

Of Molds and Mites

applaud, but when our food is so attacked and beloved objects grow green with mildew we curse. When the fungi ferment our beer and wine and age our cheese we are grateful, but when they attack our granaries we declare war on them. Thus the fungi are both blessed and despised. We cannot do without them, but they cost us much.

The fungi, of which, in all probability, there are over 100,000 species, come in two fundamental forms, the yeast that grows as single cells and reproduces either by central cell division or by budding and the hyphae which are composed of branching filaments called mycelia and which commonly bear the fruiting bodies, the spores. The hyphae may reproduce either sexually or asexually, and often both.

The fungi are a division of the plant subkingdom, the Thallophyta, and are generally classified as follows:

1. *Oomycetes*—the downy mildews which affect grasses and such crops as grapes and onions. They like to send forth their countless spores in dry, windy weather.

2. *Zygomycetes*—the molds which grow green on bread left about a little too long. An aquatic version can decimate the fish bowl, which is one reason they are called the seaweed fungi as well as the bread-mold fungi. In contrast to the oomycetes, they favor dampness and wet weather, using moisture to propagate their kind rather than going airborne.

3. *Ascomycetes*—these include the yeasts and a number of black and blue-green molds that we commonly see. They often grow on plant stems and leaves, showing up as small, mysteriously appearing circles that invariably give gardening enthusiasts fits. They also grow in the soil, and some species reach a comparatively mammoth size, such as the highly prized truffles and the morels. A good many of our life-saving antibiotics are derived from this class.

4. *Basidiomycetes*—these are the rusts and smuts of the grain fields, the puffballs kids delight to kick into small explosions of black dust, and even some of the mushrooms that gourmets seek, as well as some mushroom types they would do better to leave strictly alone.

5. *Fungi imperfecti* or *Deuteromycetes*—in this large group reside the most potently allergenic fungi, among which are the Alternaria. This prolific species casts its spores into the air everywhere in the United States except on the West Coast, where Hormodendrum takes the honor of being most rampant in its sex life. Many of the fungi imperfecti are parasitic and the cause of a good deal of disease in plants, animals, and humans. Oddly enough, some

forms actually capture tiny animals, mostly microscopic, although some species attack small worms. This particular fungi forms rings, and when a worm worms its way through, these rings inflate sharply, squeezing the worm and holding it, while other parts of the fungi's mycelium penetrate and digest the unfortunate victim.

Fungi are hardy. Although they thrive at temperatures of 70 to 90°F, some can endure subfreezing temperatures and will remain dormant until thawed out. They can then thrive once more. Intense heat, however, can be the fungi's nemesis, as can excessive dryness. In fact, for some fungi, moisture is not only necessary for growth, but also for dispensing the spores to ensure future generations. Thus rain and fog are often periods of fungi population explosions.

Those fungi that send their spores airborne keep allergists busy throughout much of the year. In northern areas fungi do have a season that runs approximately from May to October and usually peaks in July. July in many parts of the country can be a very moldy month. Unfortunately, spring and summer prevailing winds also bring spores up from the somewhat fungiladen South, where some fungi flourish the year around. Thus the fungisensitive inhabitant of northern climes often receives a double-barrelled spore shot. He or she wouldn't, however, fare any better in the South, with its spore production peaking in late summer and fall but more or less hanging in there a good part of the rest of the year.

Weather not only affects spore production and dispersion, but also the distances spores can travel. Hurricanes, gales, and tornadoes all spread spores far and wide and high into the atmosphere. High-flying spores have been found at altitudes of 16,000 feet. Since on a windless day it takes some spores several hours to drop just 100 feet, the reader can judge how long after such weather disturbances spores can remain in the air.

Environment, in addition to weather and climate, influences not only the fungi but also their impact on human health. Forest fungi differ from those of grass and cropland, whereas fungi fecundity may depend on what sort of plant life exists in any given region. In turn, a good deal of allergic rhinitis and asthma, depends on that factor of fungi fecundity. Inhaled mold spores frequently cause both these problems, and they may even be the cause of conjunctivitis, that inflamed, red-eyed condition sometimes mistaken by the uninformed as a sign of too much partying. Mold-produced conjunctivitis is difficult to treat and generally responds poorly. Contacted mold can cause dermatitis in some hypersensitive individuals, and ingested mold may produce respiratory and skin symptoms as well as gastrointestinal disturbances. Nor is this a toxic reaction such as occurs when one makes a mistake in picking mushrooms.

Fungi inhabit factories and farms as well as homes and the great out-of-doors. Outdoors, the allergic may encounter fungi in forests in rotting logs and stumps, among the leaves on the lawn, in the garden compost pile. He or she may bring mold into the house on a Christmas tree cut a bit too early or on flowers or potted plants. He or she may find it thriving in the cellar or crawl space. It makes its home in the mattress or upholstered furniture or humidifier and air conditioner. It can even dwell on paint, wallpaper paste, wood, leather, and other various fibers. It may contaminate food such as bread, or it may be deliberately invited into food as an essential ingredient such as in beer. (For an extended list of yeast-containing foods and mold-control measures, see Appendix A.) It should be noted that cheese lovers who happen to be allergic to the antibiotic penicillin need not fear cheeses aged with penicillium mold, such as Camembert or Roquefort, unless they happen to be allergic also to inhaled penicillium spores. Allergy to the antibiotic penicillin, incidentally, is a fairly prevalent allergy, one that should always be taken seriously. We discuss it in more detail in a later chapter on drug allergy.

Anyone allergic to molds should also be aware that they can reach fearsome proportions in buildings newly opened in the spring after being closed over the winter season. Those who are hypersensitive to the fungi should not rush to enter summer cabins and resort hotels and motels early in the season.

In grain-growing parts of the nation, rusts and smuts literally fill the summer air and are especially heavy at harvest time when the threshers are churning across the fields. It has been estimated that 5 million such spores can fall on every square foot of soil and that one wheat kernel can contain as many as 6 to 9 million spores. Figures such as these tend to make one feel all but buried alive by the sheer exuberance of the fungi's reproductive efforts.

In addition to that of threshing grain, there are many occupations in which workers suffer particularly heavy exposure to molds with the possibility of suffering extrinsic allergic alveolitis or, as it is more commonly called, fungal hypersensitivity pneumonitis, an asthmalike disease characterized by fever (often chronic and low grade), bronchitis, asthma, and pneumonia. Farmer's lung, resulting usually from exposure to moldy hay or grain, is one type, and mushroom workers may suffer similarly from the molds residing in the compost employed so liberally to raise these delicacies. Even lumbermen, whose occupation would seem excessively healthy if not without hazard, may be at risk from molds in infected maple tree bark. Cheese-washer's lung is caused by penicillium molds, bagassosis by molds encountered in the handling of bagasse, and sequoiosis from molds in sawdust. These same kinds of molds can inhabit air conditioners, dehumidifiers, and humidifiers to affect office workers, factory workers, hotel guests, and families in their homes.

To find out what species of molds exist in the home or workplace, petri dishes with suitable cultures much beloved by the fungi are set out in various areas. After the molds have been given sufficient time to set up residence in the dishes, they are collected and examined both for the species present and for some estimate of quantity. The dishes also serve as visible proof of a hitherto usually unseen cause for illness in the family or among workers.

How to wipe out molds?

There are fungicides on the market that are effective, but ordinary chlorine bleach does an excellent job in many areas, depending on the mode of application that is required.

Mites, like molds, are ubiquitous Arachnids. They are members of the order Ascari. Their cousins are the spiders, ticks, scorpions, and daddy long-legs. There are some 50,000 different species of mites spread across the earth, and although the giants of the mite world may be a half inch in length, the dwarfs are invisible to the naked eye.

Several species of the latter may be rampant under our own roofs, with us totally ignorant of their presence. It is not my intention here to horrify anyone, but in all probability the dust in our homes is heavily inhabited. These tiny, invisible mites are aptly called house-dust mites. They not only live in abundance, alive and thriving within our walls, but their carcasses and excrement float about to fill our lungs, resulting in rhinitis and/or asthma for the hypersensitive, for they are potent allergens.

Thus what may have been considered as inorganic "dirt" could be very much alive or, at the very least, once alive, and organic in good part. Because it is so laden with organic matter, house dust differs essentially from outside dirt, which is basically inorganic. Although the latter may act as an irritant in our respiratory systems, the former acts as both irritant and allergen. If looked at too closely, house dust can prove to be an unpleasant mixture of dead and alive mites, their excrement, dead and alive bacteria, human and animal dander (skin scales and scurf shed by just about all members of the animal kingdom, including ourselves), plant and food remnants, kapok and cotton linters from deteriorating furniture, rugs, mattresses, and the like plus the molds that dwell within—enough to send anyone for mop and pail! Small

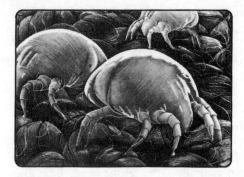

D. pteronyssinus, the household dust mite. Photo courtesy of Fisons Corporation.

wonder so many of us sniffle and sneeze and wheeze, for much of this composite dust swirls about in the air and is highly allergenic. A good deal of attention, especially in Europe and England, has recently focused on the house-dust mite as being the main cause of a good deal of allergy, rhinitis and asthma especially.

There are several potently allergenic species of these mites, officially called Dermatophagoides. Apparently various regions of the world harbor their own particular dominant species. Europe, for instance, has one type; we have another. One Japanese study uncovered 35 different species of mites in the dust of a Japanese household, a statistic that would surely unnerve anyone.

Mites appear to be particularly fond of colonizing mattresses, carpets, and overstuffed furniture. They can also be found in quantity in stuffed toys, and if one were to look under the bed with a microscope, the scene would be devastating. Significantly smaller populations turn up in hospital bedding, perhaps because of more frequent and energetic cleaning methods plus the use of plastic covers, for this last procedure apparently drastically cuts down mite populations. Nevertheless, hospitals are not exempt.

There also appear to be seasonal fluctuations in mite populations. An English study demonstrated that mite colonies were smaller on mattresses during the winter, but exploded in size during the late spring and summer.

It has also been discovered that the house-dust mite consists mainly of water, in fact, about 81% water, and it is thus exquisitely sensitive to the whims of humidity. If the weather turns hot and dry, the mite loses about 46.5% of its moisture, and it will die. This finding has led to the suggestion that to get rid of mites in mattresses and the like they should be subjected periodically to a high, dry heating procedure. This somewhat drastic measure might be practical for hospitals and other institutions but hardly seems manageable for the average home.

That the house-dust mite stands high on the list of potent allergens has been demonstrated repeatedly. In one study of 544 asthmatic patients who registered positive reactions to skin prick tests, 82% indicated positive results to the house-dust or acarine mite, whereas 66% demonstrated allergy to pollen, 38% to animal dander, 16% to foods, 16% to Aspergillus fumigatus, and 21% to other molds. Many of these patients obviously suffered from hypersensitivity to several allergens, which is often the case.

There has been one report in the literature of a fatal bronchial asthma attack attributed to house-dust allergy. A teenage boy who had suffered from asthma was apparently well controlled when his home was kept as free of dust as was humanly possible. For two years his symptoms had abated, but in a stay at a school he suffered an attack of status asthmaticus, a severe and continuous asthma attack that can be life-threatening. In this case, it was fatal. It was concluded that he had been exposed at the school to dust allergens.

Trying to rid the home of the house-dust mite is anything but easy. Chemical measures have not yet proved practical, since they must be applied to beds and other furniture for some duration before becoming effective and this procedure may be as hazardous to humans as to mites. Also, mites seem to be resistant to all but the most powerful substances. Researchers have been working on biological controls and have found a mite predator, C. eruditus, which preys on various species of the house-dust mite. The jungle code of red of tooth and claw may be going on invisibly at one's feet!

The best of all ways to rid the home of dust and the house-dust mite is outlined in Appendix B. These measures admittedly require effort, but they are effective. And now that the reader is aware that the dust ball rolling across the floor toward his or her feet may well harbor a colony of countless tiny beings which can affect the nasal and bronchial structures as well as one's general health, perhaps such measures will seem well worth that effort.

GLOSSARY

Hyphae: tubular filaments which form the mycelia of fungi.

Mycelia: the vegetative part of the fungi.

Thallophyta: simple plants without roots, stems or leaves; that is, the fungi and algae.

Spore: an asexual reproductive cell which can develop an adult without fusion with another cell.

Hypersensitivity pneumonitis: a respiratory condition characterized by bronchitis, asthma, inflammation of the smaller subdivisions of the bronchi, and pneumonia.

Arachnids: a class of Arthropods (invertebrate animals with jointed legs and segmented bodies) lacking wings and antennae.

Acarina: a division of Arachnids containing mites.

Dermatophagoides: a genus of Acarina containing house-dust mites.

SUMMARY

1. Molds and mites are ubiquitous and potent allergens.
2. Fungi can cause disease in humans as parasites or as allergens.
3. There are five types of fungi:

    Oomycetes

    Zygomycetes

    Ascomycetes

    Basidiomycetes

    Fungi Imperfecti: the species containing members that are most potently allergenic

4. Most fungi reproduce by spore formation.
5. Factors such as weather, climate, humidity, and wind influence both the production and dispersion of fungi.
6. Mites are also both parasitic and allergenic.
7. The house-dust mite is also ubiquitous and a potent allergen.
8. Low humidity and high temperatures can be a house-dust mite's undoing, since the water content of its body is extremely high and it cannot tolerate desiccation.
9. Control measures for dust are the most effective way to rid the home of house-dust mites (and other inhalant allergens).

six

A man's house may be his castle, but it may also be his affliction. I am not talking about the mortgage here, but of the well-known fact that accidents occurring in the home are a leading cause of injury and death, plus what we have just discussed, the problems molds and mites can provoke within the sanctuary of one's four walls. Unfortunately, those tiny motes dancing in a beam of sunlight falling upon the floor contain a variety of other substances, some of which are also allergens, some of which are irritants, and some of which are probably neither but just plain dirt.

If we were to enter a more-or-less typical American home, perhaps the first thing we would see would be a large, long-haired cat curled up comfortably in an armchair, obviously its favorite napping spot if one can judge by the slight mat of hair on the cushions. The cat is handsome and very clean, but . . . as we have noted, all animals, including ourselves, shed dander—skin scales and scurf—into the air. Cat dander is especially potently allergenic, in part, perhaps, because it is particularly light and airy. It floats about freely and is difficult to corral. It may even affect the allergic individual for days

Also in the Air

after the cat has been removed from the scene. The cat's hide has an affinity also for all sorts of other allergens to add to its own. And cat saliva may contain a unique allergen, which, when the cat washes itself and the saliva dries, may be added to the rest of the output.

About one in four allergic patients exhibit positive reactions to skin tests for cat and dog dander. Unfortunately, they tend to react somewhat drastically to cat dander. I have had patients who need only enter a room through one door after the cat has exited from another to suddenly swell about the eyes, itch around eyes, nose, and mouth, and suffer an abrupt attack of wheezing.

Incidentally, the cat sensitive have more than house cats to worry about. Such people would do well to detour around the lion house at the zoo, forgo leopard-skin coats, and do without tiger-skin rugs. Cat hair can find its way on occasion into toys, gloves, slippers, furniture (upholstered), bathrobes, and caps. If it is thoroughly cleaned and treated, its potency is dimmed somewhat, but even so, anyone who suffers a severe allergy to cats should bypass such items. Studies conducted to determine whether different breeds of cats are more potently allergenic than others suggest that the Siamese cat is the chief offender.

Dogs are next in line as a prime animal cause of allergy, perhaps because almost all of us possess at least one of them in the home. Oddly enough, dogs of different breeds, although they share common allergens, may put forth a special brand of their own. The result is that some people are allergic to one particular breed but may be able to tolerate dogs of other breeds.

Dogs and cats within the family are a tremendous asset. Dogs help guard the premises against intruders, and cats keep mice out of the kitchen, but most of all, they are treasured companions and an invaluable way to teach children compassion and responsibility, the former a gift not to be taken lightly in our somewhat violent society. Thus when someone in the family turns up allergic to the family pet or pets, we have a situation that is somewhere between a rock and a hard place. The anguish can be very real and deep, and sometimes that anguish must be weighed against the severity of the allergy involved. The mildly allergic, for instance, may be able to tolerate the pet if it resides in the backyard and makes infrequent forays into the house. But for the severely allergic, especially for the asthmatic, there is really no choice. It is possible the pet could reside totally in the backyard, but if the allergy problem persisted, the pet should go to another good home.

For children and, I suspect, for a good many adults as well, saying goodbye to a beloved pet can be traumatic. Parents of a child who find themselves in such a fix should do their best to soften the separation, although there is really no easy way to take a pet from a child. The best a parent can do is to concoct a believable and gentle tale about the pet going off to get married and to have a family of its own, or, like Charlie Brown's Snoopy, going off to visit the mother he hasn't seen since puppyhood or kittenhood, as the case may be. Even so, this can be a family tragedy, but when it is weighed against the possibilities of chronic, disabling, debilitating, and sometimes fatal asthma, the deed must be done.

Sometimes a new pet can be substituted. Not, of course, anything with fur or feathers, which pretty much leaves the choice to fish or reptiles. Such pets may leave something to be desired as far as loveability is concerned, but they can be interesting. I had one young asthmatic patient whose mother really went beyond the call of duty to provide her son with a pet he could call his own. When I jokingly suggested a snake, the boy seized upon it and asked for one for Christmas. I am not certain exactly what the parents thought of me, for it took a little doing to find a pet shop that dealt in snakes, but one was finally unearthed some distance from their home town. They decided that this snake, a docile boa constrictor, was just the thing. However, the day they were to pick it up was cold, and the boa is a tropical being. If it were to survive the trip home, it had to be kept very warm. My young patient's mother solved the problem as few women and, I venture, few men would have cared to do. She wrapped the snake around her waist under her overcoat and home they came. Surely, this is mother courage at its best!

Many a youngster has yearned for a pony on his way to adulthood, but, unfortunately, if he or she is allergic, horse dander can be potent. Parents should also be aware that horsey clothes and boots can bring the dander into the house. They should also be aware that horse dander is antigenically similar to horse serum, so that the person allergic to the dander should be careful about receiving horse antisera in immunizations such as those for tetanus or in antivenom such as that for black-widow spider bites.

Down on the farm, the allergic farmer and/or allergic members of his family may have difficulty with all sorts of animal danders or feathers. Even the relatively hairless pig puts out a potent supply. Off the farm, animal hair and hides are employed in a number of household goods and items of clothing. Rugs, furniture, even toys may contain horse hair, and, of course, coats and sweaters may employ material from cats to cattle, sheep to seals, rabbits to minks. Feathers are highly allergenic, and whoever is allergic to them must forego the pleasures of down comforters and feather pillows. Nor should there be a canary or parakeet or bird of any description in the house.

It may appear that the hypersensitive individual is at the mercy of a world full of things guaranteed to make him or her miserable. Unfortunately, we are not done yet with the list of potentially baneful substances that could be in the air he or she must breathe. There is, for instance, cottonseed, which is so potent an allergen that allergists are cautious in testing for sensitivity to it, since a simple skin test with an extract of the material can provoke a severe reaction in some patients. Cotton linters, which often contain the seed to some degree, are used to stuff toys, furniture, cushions, and comforters. In this form, the cotton can provoke allergy, whereas cotton sheets and clothing made from long cotton fibers with the seed ginned out are not allergenic.

Cotton linters and cottonseed are commonly found in the following products:

Doughnuts and other bakery items	Candles
Candies	Carpets
Lining of coats and jackets	Rope
Lining of underwear	Fertilizers
Photographic film	Animal feeds
Some dyes	

In the process of manufacture, heat makes cottonseed oil used in margarine, paint, furniture polish, salves, and linaments less potent, although for the severely allergic, it can still kick up symptoms if inhaled or ingested.

Flaxseed, generally employed in linseed oil or in meal, is also a fairly potent allergen. It may be found in the following:

Roman meal	Insulation
Hair-setting lotion	Laxatives
Animal feed	Fertilizer
Cough medicine	Paint
Depilatories	

Orris root, which once was commonly employed as a base for cosmetics, produced so much rhinitis and asthma that the cosmetic industry curtailed its use. However, it may still be in such things as bath salts, toothpastes, and powders, perfumes, and hair tonics. Derived from plants of the iris family, it was valuable for cosmetics because it not only retained its pleasant violet odor, but could retain other scents as well.

Pyrethrum, which shares a common allergen with ragweed and sage, is frequently found in insecticides. It can affect those who are allergic to these other members of the botanical family Compositae.

Castor bean can be a potent allergen, but fortunately its use is not pervasive, although it is in some cosmetics, fertilizers, and laxatives. Jute, once widely employed in ropes and burlap bags before the advent of nylon and plastics, can still cause asthma when used in rug pads in the home.

The vegetable gums—karaya, acacia, and tragacanth—are widely employed in a variety of unlikely goods, and if inhaled or ingested, they can cause problems for the allergic. They can be found in some hair-setting lotions and some toothpastes, salad dressing and ice cream, pie fillings, and in adhesives. Anyone allergic to them will have to be wary, for they tend to show up in surprising products.

Speaking of adhesives, those who are allergic to fish will have to avoid fish glues in all likelihood, since these, too, can be potent allergens. Building model planes may not be the thing for some allergic children, and it is possible that such glue in bookbindings, labels, furniture, and paper boxes could provoke symptoms. The odor of fish glue can also be an irritant and can act as a trigger for rhinitis and/or asthma even though the individual is not allergic to the glue itself. Strong odors such as those of wood fires and tobacco smoke, moth balls, fresh newsprint, even gasoline may also act in this fashion by irritating the respiratory system and thus precipitating an allergic reaction. Allergists have even indicted cooking foods of being such triggers, especially odors of frying foods such as fish and eggs.

One of the firmest arguments for segregating smokers in public places and of making smoking in enclosed public conveyances such as elevators illegal is that tobacco smoke is a health hazard to all who must breathe it, and this is especially so for people who suffer respiratory allergies, particularly those who have asthma. Asthma patients who are smokers themselves do so at their own risk, but it seems hardly just that those who refrain for the sake of their health must suffer because others fill the air they must breathe with smoke.

Recent studies suggest that tobacco and tobacco smoke are more than irritants, that they can, in fact, sensitize to cause allergic reactions. Definitive proof, however, waits in the wings, and the problem is complicated by the presence in tobacco products of pesticide traces and the like.

Mammals and plants are not the only suppliers of allergens afloat, for insects shed an incredible amount of debris into the air, most of which is so minute that it goes unnoticed. Wing scales, bits of chitlin, discarded and disintegrating cocoons and webs (often covered with dust), and feces make up a goodly proportion of aerial pollution. Two species in particular, the caddis fly and the mayfly, shed enormous amounts of material in some regions of the United States, especially in the neighborhood of the Great Lakes. These insects appear as adults at specific times and in huge numbers. Starting in July the mayflies appear in waves of hundreds of thousands of insects. They take to the air before shedding their final skins, which can then be found clinging to buildings and trees or scattered over the ground. Unfortunately from the mayfly's point of view, but fortunately for the allergic, the insect lives for only a few hours, at most for a day or two. Its final function is to mate and for the female to lay her eggs and then die. Thus, during these incredible swarms carcasses may cover the sidewalks and porches of the lake and river towns where the mayflies breed. Things can actually get slippery underfoot, and people have the somewhat unpleasant task of sweeping up and of disposing of the remains.

The story of the caddis fly is similar, and both insects can cause quite a bit of allergy in the final hours of their lives.

The unpleasant cockroach can also cause considerable discomfort for the allergic, not only because it, too, sheds debris and feces into the air, but also because it has a nasty habit of vomiting partially digested food all over the place, including over any human edibles that it can get to.

Even a few beekeepers have had to give up their profession, not because they were allergic to bee venom, although that also happens on occasion, but because they were hypersensitive to bee dust, which, I suppose, must be considerable in and around the hives.

Air pollution, which has become a recognized fact of our industrial lives these last 30 years, can greatly aggravate, if not cause, allergy diseases, especially asthma. The asthma patient generally has been the first affected during many of the air-pollution episodes that have plagued the industrial nations. Even if not hypersensitive to pollutant particles in the air, the asthmatic's respiratory system is unstable and can be vulnerable to irritants. In the Thanksgiving 1966 New York City air-pollution episode, it is estimated that for seven days, an additional 24 people more than the statistical daily average died each day in the city's hospitals, most of them victims of severe asthma. During the infamous Donora, Pennsylvania, pollution crisis of 1948, it was estimated that 90% of those who were asthmatics were affected by the pollutants in the smog versus 40% of those of the total population. A group of researchers studied Philadelphia school children a few years ago and discovered that three times as many attacks of asthma occurred on days when the pollution index was high and nine times as many occurred when high pollution was coupled with a rise in barometric pressure.

We are often given to looking back in nostalgia to the days before leaf burning was banned in many cities and towns. Those small bright fires in the gutters or on the lawn signaled the cool, clear days of late fall and heralded the coming of winter. Sight and smell were mighty pleasant. Nostalgia aside, the smell, at least, was hazardous to some, for the pungent smoke could irritate nasal and lung tissue, with the result that the susceptible respiratory system of the asthmatic frequently reacted with wheezing and obstruction. To compound the problem, no doubt, a good many fungal spores were also released as the leaves were raked and piled.

Irritant or allergen, there is more afloat than meets the eye!

GLOSSARY

Dander: tiny particles as from skin, feathers, or hair, that may cause allergies.

Irritant: an agent producing local inflammation.

SUMMARY

1. Animal dander, especially of cats, dogs, and horses, and feathers are potent allergens.

2. Other allergens frequently inhaled are:

Cottonseed	Karaya
Pyrethrum	Wood smoke
Castor bean	Kapok
Acacia	Tobacco smoke
Flaxseed	Tragacanth
Fish glue	Cooking odors

3. Tobacco smoke, wood smoke, cooking odors, burning leaves, air pollutants can all be irritants as well as allergens.

4. Insect debris shed into the air can also be potently allergenic.

seven

We physicians give out all sorts of good advice, and we are very fond of parroting such sayings as, "You should eat to live, not live to eat." "You are what you eat." We are quite right, of course, for obesity is a high-priority American problem, and poor nutrition may be a close second. Food can have other ill effects. It can be contaminated by bacteria, or it may contain toxic substances, or the ingestor could be either intolerant or hypersensitive to it or to substances added to it during processing.

Food poisoning needs no explanation, I suspect, since the chicken salad at a church function that sends its participants in droves to the hospital is a well-known if unfortunate phenomenon. Happily, such incidents usually turn out all right with no permanent harm done, although there may be a universal dislike henceforth for chicken salad. Much grimmer are the accounts of botulism from such foods as inadequately canned beans. There may even be the occasional strangeness of a tale such as that of the Northwest Coast Indians who bury whole salmon in the beaches, then dig them up weeks later when they are fully "ripe." Considered a gourmet delight, if botulism has settled in, the treat may be the diner's last.

Perfectly Good Food?

Foods sometimes contain somewhat toxic substances naturally which may be neutralized in their preparation. Lima beans, for instance, may cause intolerance symptoms if served up undercooked. Foods may also take up substances from the soil or water in amounts that can be toxic. Nitrates, lead, and mercury arrive in this manner on the dining room table. Some vegetables grown on truck farms bordering the New Jersey Turnpike, for example, have been found to contain high lead levels on occasion. Cattle who have grazed on a pasture that was once an old apple orchard have produced arsenic traces in their milk from their consumption of grass grown in soil heavily laced by old arsenic sprays. Perhaps even stranger, undiscriminating bees may gather pollen from toxic plants and confer the poison to whomever consumes the honey. And cows who dine on white snake root may make whoever drinks their milk thoroughly miserable. As a matter of fact, this last problem can be a serious matter for children.

One odd case of food poisoning occurred not long ago in a Tennessee family when they consumed tomatoes grown on a plant someone had cleverly grafted to a jimsonweed root and lower stem. Although the news account of this incident did not indicate whether family members developed a "high" from the stramoium alkaloids the tomatoes absorbed from the jimsonweed, they definitely made them ill.

Fungi can transform perfectly good food into potent poisons. I suppose that the best known example is that of ergot, for ergot in rye once periodically decimated whole villages in Europe. Symptoms caused by this toxic transformation could be horrendous, with victims frequently exhibiting gangrene of the extremities, especially of the fingers and toes, and of nervous system manifestations such as itching and tingling of the skin, mental loss, deafness, and dimmed vision.

Some foods are capable of causing the release of histamine, which, of course, would be the last thing an allergic person needs. Such foods—shellfish, strawberries, egg white—should be avoided when the hypersensitive individual is suffering symptoms, especially of hay fever and eczema. These foods could be the proverbial straws to break the camel's back.

Some spices, nutmeg is a good example, may cause uncomfortable symptoms of intolerance if ingested to excess.

In this age of pill-popping there is also a problem of synergism between some drugs and some foods. For example, a variety of tranquilizers and central nervous system drugs combined with foods that contain tryamine can produce toxic effects which can be severe, even fatal. Psychotropic drugs that contain monoamine oxidase are especially dangerous in this regard, and the result of this combination can be a hypertensive crisis. Tryamine is a pressor amine, a nitrogenous substance capable of raising blood pressure. Foods that contain it are as follows:

Aged cheeses, especially Cheddar   Figs

Chicken livers   Pods of broad beans

Pickled herring   Red wine

Some beers   Champagne

Most of these problems with food we consider more or less as natural and certainly apart from an interference from us. We are great meddlers, however, which is often a good thing, but is also sometimes a terrible misfortune. When it comes to food, we like to think that we can improve on Nature. So we tinker, removing a good bit of what she puts in and adding what we consider appropriate at the moment. All sorts of substances get tossed into the pot—artificial colors and flavors; things to pep up, smooth out, fill up; chemicals to add months to a normal shelf life of a few weeks. All these are called intentional additives, and they can affect us as either toxic substances or allergens. In the former case, it is decidedly unsettling to see them being removed by the FDA after years of being served up in our diet. In the latter case, a good many allergic people react both to aspirin and to a yellow dye that is commonly employed in a number of food products. This dye, tartrazine, although chemically different, is somewhat similar to the salicylate of aspirin, and allergy to either is not only quite common but can be severe. It is quite simple to refrain from consuming aspirin, but it is far more difficult to avoid tartrazine (FD&C Yellow No. 5). The following partial list of foods and other ingestants which could contain tartrazine will serve to demonstrate just how difficult:

Beer

Tea

Lunch meats

Candies

Gum

Toothpaste

Ice cream

Jams and jellies

Oleomargarine

Bakery goods (except bread)

Gin

Soft drinks

Hot dogs

Cake mixes

Wine

Mouthwash

Oil of wintergreen

Artificial colors and flavors have come in for special criticism not only because they seem an unnecessary addition to perfectly good food but also because they seem to have the most far-reaching effects on health with, perhaps, the exception of the nitrites. Some physicians attribute at least some of the hyperactivity in children that is apparently on the increase in our land to the abundant use of these coal-tar dyes and chemical flavors. Children consume a goodly quantity of highly colored, highly flavored products, and although the claim that such additives contribute to aberrant behavior is disputed, there is surely some validity to the theory that some of these substances do cause allergic reactions in the nervous system, which, in turn, may lead to emotional and behavioral disturbances of one kind or another. And even as the notion of childhood hyperactivity is pooh-poohed, up pops another claim that "junk foods" may be responsible in part for some of the increasing incidence of violent crime.

Whatever the eventual outcome of these claims and counterclaims, allergists are aware that some additives do affect both health and behavior. A case in point is monosodium glutamate, which has been indicted as the cause of Chinese-restaurant syndrome, an unhappy sequel to an enjoyable Chinese dinner for some individuals. Complaints usually include headache, weakness, a sense of numbness, and heart palpitations. In a later chapter we explore a somewhat astonishing list of similar allergic reactions of the central nervous system and their sometimes bizarre consequences.

Unintentional additives also find their way to American tables as residues of pesticides sprayed on crops or of drugs fed to animals to enhance weight gain and to prevent diseases, which can occur when large-scale animal-factory methods are employed. An example so well known that preschool children probably know all about it is the story of DDT. It is believed that almost every American now has some DDT stored in his or her body fat, most of which arrived there via the food chain. For some people this can still be a worrisome problem, even though DDT use has been banned a number of years. Just recently it was discovered that the entire population of a small Alabama town, located downstream from a chemical plant that manufactured DDT for a good many years, have extremely high body levels of the pesticide. Unfortunately for them, DDT from the plant heavily polluted the streams and, in turn, the fish on which most of the townspeople depended for subsistence. What the eventual effects of such high levels of DDT will be is uncertain; nobody really knows. Certain chemical substances we have incorporated into ourselves in our technological society could be time bombs ticking away until the day the timing mechanism suddenly runs out. DDT may be one of them.

Another area of concern about unintentional additives is that of the widespread and heavy use of antibiotics in meat animals, for such usage encourages the development of resistant bacteria. The result is that when such bacteria infect humans, wonder drugs are no longer effective. The great medical breakthrough they once represented could be cancelled completely.

Thus foods can have various health effects other than those due to allergy. The physician, therefore, must consider a plenitude of possibilities before settling on allergy. Cow's milk, for all its fine reputation as a perfect food, can pose several disturbing problems. There is, for instance, a condition due to lactase deficiency which is quite common among peoples of other than Northern European heritage. The reason suggested for this disparity in the possession of the lactase enzyme is that those populations who took up dairying evolved the ability to produce sufficient lactase in the gastrointestinal tract to tolerate milk, whereas those folks who did not keep cows, and thus did not use milk, never developed enough lactase to break down the lactose content of milk. The result of lactase deficiency is gastrointestinal disorders, with primary symptoms of diarrhea, bloating, and general discomfort. This malabsorption problem does not extend to some milk products, such as certain aged cheeses and yogurt, for in these products the lactose is broken down by bacteria or fungi.

Celiac disease is another problem the physician must consider in young children who develop gastrointestinal disorders. It is generally first seen in youngsters from ages of six months to six years and is characterized by a failure to thrive, poor appetite, fatty stools, and muscle weakness. Most celiac patients cannot tolerate gluten that is found in wheat and other grains.

Cystic fibrosis must also be ruled out before allergy can be ruled in.

This tragic disease of the young, with its poor prognosis, involves an abnormality of the exocrine glands leading to pancreatic insufficiency and chronic respiratory symptoms with an overproduction of mucus. Diagnosis is made on the basis of a number of specific tests, one of which is a sweat test, for in this disease sweat electrolytes are abnormally high.

Infection and parasitic infestation can also produce symptoms akin to those caused by gastrointestinal allergy.

When we do finally arrive at the point where we can consider that something the patient ingested is at the bottom of the problem because he or she is hypersensitive to whatever it is, we find that there are a number of symptoms he or she can display. The following list will give the reader some idea of the possibilities:

Itching, burning and edema of lips, tongue, gums

Chapped and/or inflamed lips

Rash around the mouth

Canker sores

Bad breath

An odd-looking tongue called geographical tongue

Difficulty in swallowing

Cough

Nausea and/or vomiting

Heartburn, bloating, belching

Pylorus (spasms of the opening between the stomach and duodenum)

Abdominal pain

Diarrhea and/or constipation

Blood and/or mucus in stools

Anal itching and inflammation of anus and rectum

Tenesmus (a persistent feeling that the bowel needs emptying, with resulting straining)

Allergy to food may result in an immediate reaction, the usual symptoms being hives, angioedema, and nausea and vomiting and/or diarrhea. Anaphylactic shock can occur with falling blood pressure and loss of consciousness. Foods most often responsible are milk, eggs, fish, peanuts (legumes), and nuts.

Delayed reactions can follow the ingestion of a food by hours or even days and is probably the result of absorption of the allergen from the gastro-intestinal tract into the bloodstream, where it comes into eventual contact with sensitized cells, often in other body systems. This is in contrast to an immediate reaction in which the food allergen meets the sensitized cells within the gastrointestinal system itself.

As in other allergies, several factors play an important role in whether or not sensitization and reaction occur. The size and nature of the food allergen is one such factor. The protein or carbohydrate content of the food determines to a large extent its potency as an allergen. Cow's milk, for instance, contains over 20 proteins. Of these, the most important allergens are beta lactoglobulin, alpha lactalbumin, bovine serum albumin, and casein. The first of these appears to be the most potent. In eggs it is the white with its potent allergen, ovomucoid, that is the prime offender. Fortunately, cooking can alter the allergenic potency of a food, usually decreasing it. Often, too, stale food is less allergenic than fresh. What this may mean to an allergic gourmet is an open question!

A second important factor is the duration and amount of exposure to a food. The infant on a cow's milk formula who consumes little else is rather naturally being heavily exposed to those milk allergens. During strawberry or cantaloupe season, which is so short and so sweet, the predisposed to allergy can consume too much of a good thing. For this reason the foods most often indicted in allergy are those most commonly found in the diet—milk, eggs, wheat, and corn.

The condition and efficiency of the individual's gastrointestinal tract plays an important role. It is one of the reasons why allergy to food is most common in infants and young children, for their immature gastrointestinal tracts allow penetration of more and larger protein molecules that reach IgE antibodies in the submucosa or in the vascular system. As we have noted, the gastrointestinal tract is lined with mucosa, just beneath which are the plasma cells containing the antibodies IgE, IgA, and others. Although it is thought that IgA helps block the interaction of allergens and IgE, unfor-tunately the very young usually have not developed sufficient IgA to in-terfere successfully. This does not mean that hypersensitivity to foods cannot occur at any other time of life. It can and it does, for there is always that factor of exposure to consider, which coupled with the factor of genetic predisposition is enough to make one allergic to a food at some time down the line.

Infection can also open the door to allergy, especially when the gastrointestinal tract is involved. And, since infections are more common in childhood, then so will be an allergy.

Allergy to food can be an unpredictable business. Some allergists have designated two types: a fixed allergic response and a variable or cyclical type. In the first the patient reacts to a specific food allergen with specific symptoms. Neither the amount of food involved nor the interval between exposures varies this reaction. For example, a person allergic to eggs may suffer a lifetime hypersensitivity, reacting to even a tiny amount of ingested egg with immediate symptoms of hives, angioedema, and even anaphylactic shock. Fortunately, this is the least common type, but it can be severe and sometimes very dangerous. One physician has recorded the case of a woman who was having her hair fixed in a beauty parlor and who accepted a handful of sunflower seeds from a fellow beauty seeker. She ate a few, suddenly announced that she couldn't breath, and within minutes she was dead. Although such an intense anaphylactic reaction is rare, individuals suffering this type of reaction *must* avoid the offending food or foods entirely. It has been estimated that between 5% and 10% of the food allergic fall within this risky category.

The variable or cyclical type of response to food allergens is quite different, in that reactions are generally much milder, and the patient's symptoms vary not only with the amount of the food allergen consumed but also with the interval between ingestion and symptoms. This last makes it a good deal more difficult to diagnose. However, the patient suffering this type of food allergy may be able to develop a tolerance for the offending food as long as he or she consumes it in moderate amounts at infrequent intervals. Even so, he or she must be wary of those additional factors we have discussed in an earlier chapter which make up the allergic load to challenge one's tolerance. Nor can he or she succumb to gluttony, for there is no place for overconsumption in allergy to food.

Diagnosis of food allergy can be simple or difficult. Since the patient's complaints are apt to be diffuse and somewhat nebulous, it is often the latter. Although skin tests are not as reliable as they are for inhalant allergies, they can serve to focus suspicion, as can RAST tests. Thus the allergist cannot fall back on the usual panoply of scarifiers and needles and extract jars. There are no specific laboratory tests either, other than those to rule out other possibilities. The most important diagnostic tool is the patient's history, for in this somewhat lengthy and detailed interview will lie the necessary clues nine times out of ten.

"Can't drink milk," the patient may say. "It never did agree with me, even when I was a kid." Yet, of course, he or she may be ingesting milk in dozens of foods and food products. The best way to pin down whether milk is indeed the cause of the symptoms is to remove it from the patient's diet for a few weeks, then, if symptoms are relieved, reintroduce it and see what happens. If symptoms return, milk is the offender.

However, oddly enough, the fact that a patient may say, "I love milk. I drink a quart a day every day," may also be a clue, for an inordinate liking for a food may be a sign of allergy to it in much the same vein as a pronounced dislike can be.

In general, about one in five food-allergic patients are aware of the food or foods that cause their symptoms. This is not really surprising, considering that the connection between ingesting a food and subsequent upset or other symptoms can be quite clear. Parents of very young children, for instance, should heed preferences to the extent that if a child persistently refuses a food, eggs especially, that child may be registering discomfort. Perhaps, if the parent were to look more closely, he or she might note that the child's face was flushed or was a little swollen or there was apparently a rash around the mouth, all indications of possible allergy to that food.

The other side of the coin, an addiction to the food that one is hypersensitive to, is interesting if hypothetical. It is postulated that it is akin to the mechanism that chains the alcoholic to drinks, the addict to drugs, the smoker to cigarettes. The food addict may even undergo withdrawal symptoms!

In any case, there are still four out of five patients to be diagnosed, and although inordinate likings and dislikings are helpful, they will not solve most of our mysteries. As we have noted, the allergic react most frequently to the staple foods of milk, eggs, wheat, and corn, which, unfortunately, are contained in an endless variety of food products. How to find out if it is one of these four or something much more exotic? The best of all ways to get at the crux of the food allergic's problem is to place him or her on an elimination diet. Quite simply, this is an abbreviated menu with the potent food allergens and those foods both physician and patient suspect removed from the diet. It can be somewhat spartan, but it will only be temporary, and if you happen to also suffer from obesity, you can kill two birds with one stone. A sample elimination diet might look something like this:

Breakfast   Fruit or fruit juice: pear, grapefruit, apple

                                       Ry-Krisp (plain)

	Tea
	Cooked rice or oatmeal
	Isomil (soybean milk)
Lunch	Meat: lamb, veal, or roast beef
	Vegetable: carrots, beets, lettuce, asparagus, squash
	Tea
	Ry-Krisp (plain)
	Isomil
	Fruit as at breakfast
Dinner	Meat as at lunch
	Vegetables as at lunch
	Tea
	Ry-Krisp
	Isomil
	Fruit as at lunch

The patient will not starve on this menu, but, of course, it will do nothing for the gourmet. However, each elimination diet must be especially tailored to the patient involved. It may not be quite so spartan, although some allergists believe in eliminating everything except spring water and Ry-Krisp.

Whatever the regimen, the patient is asked to maintain it for a period of 14 to 18 days, long enough, that is, to clear the body of any lingering food allergens. Usually, by the end of this period all allergy symptoms will have vanished also, but if not, the physician will have to tinker further and remove whatever other foods remain in the diet.

But let us say that the patient is now symptom free and the elimination diet has done its thing. We then begin to add foods back into the menu one at a time, with enough time elapsed between each addition to allow symptoms to appear if they are going to. Each food that is added should be eaten every day for an optimum period of four days, with the food served up twice a day if possible and the patient can stand it. The idea is to really challenge the patient with each food returned to the diet. I must add here that, of course, any food that has caused a severe reaction should never be readded. That food is best avoided if not forever, for at least a year or more, and then only attempted in small amounts (never if the reaction was anaphylactic in nature) and in the safety of the physician's office.

If symptoms do recur, the food is once again eliminated from the diet, then tried once more in a month's time. If symptoms recur three times after that particular food is eaten, then it is safe to say that it is the cause of the patient's woes. The patient should then avoid it entirely for a number of months or a year, then, if the reaction is not an immediate or "fixed" reaction, he or she may be able to tolerate it once again, but only in moderation and infrequently.

I supply my patients with a copy of instructions for an elimination diet that you will find in Appendix D. I must emphasize that this is no do-it-yourself procedure. Like any other special diet, it should be under the supervision of a physician, for what boots it to discover what is causing one's allergy only to lose one's general health in the process? Besides, foods come in botanical plant families, so that a patient may cross-react to a second food. For example, if an individual is allergic to peas, he or she may also be allergic to peanuts, for they both belong to the legume plant family. It is possible also to have problems with soybeans, for they, too, are legumes. Anyone who is allergic to mustard should approach cabbage and cauliflower with some caution. And if almonds cause a problem, so may peaches and prunes. Fortunately, cross-reactivity is not common. For a longer list of common food families, see Appendix E.

A far more common problem are hidden foods in food products, for they are not always specifically named on the label. For example, *vegetable oil* does not identify whether it is peanut oil or cottonseed, and corn syrup may be the sweetener in many products rather than cane sugar. Foods like potato chips and doughnuts may be fried in one kind of oil at one time and in another a few months later, depending, I suppose, on current prices and supply.

It is easy to see that food allergy can be a real trial for the individual whose allergy is more than mild and who reacts to the staple foods.

GLOSSARY

Tryamine: a pressor amine, a nitrogenous substance capable of raising blood pressure.

Synergism: The interaction of two substances to produce an effect greater than could be produced by either alone.

Lactase deficiency: a deficiency of the enzyme lactase, which breaks down the lactose of cow's milk in the gastrointestinal tract into more digestible components.

Celiac disease: a chronic intestinal disorder characterized by a failure to thrive, fatty stools, and muscle weakness.

Fixed reaction: reaction of specific symptoms to a specific food.

Variable or *cyclical reaction:* symptoms vary with exposure as does the interval between exposure and symptoms.

Elimination diet: a diet devoid of potent allergenic foods and those suspected of causing allergy in a specific patient.

SUMMARY

1. Foods may cause health problems in a number of ways:

　　When contaminated by bacteria

　　When containing toxic substances

　　When interacting with certain drugs

　　When allergenic for a hypersensitive individual

2. Intentional additives are natural and synthetic substances incorporated into various foods to color, flavor, preserve, blend, fill, smooth, thicken, and the like.

3. Unintentional additives are residues of pesticides, drugs, and soil contaminants that find their way into the food more or less accidentally.

4. Differential diagnosis must rule out illnesses such as cystic fibrosis and celiac disease, enzyme deficiencies, parasitic infestations, and infections before ruling allergy to food in.

5. Allergic reactions to food can be immediate or delayed, with the former generally more severe and more difficult to control except by complete avoidance of the offending food.

6. A number of factors are involved in allergy to food:

Nature of the allergen

Amount and duration of exposure

Presence of allergic-load factors

Condition and efficiency of the individual's gastrointestinal tract

Genetic predisposition

7. An elimination diet based on the patient's history in the main is usually the best method of uncovering the offending food.

eight

A dispassionate observer might conclude that we moderns think of ourselves as giant test tubes into which we continually pour various chemicals. And always hopefully. For we take our medications seriously, to solve not only our health problems but the problems of our souls as well. Physicians prescribe and people buy over the counter a bewildering array of drugs to heal, to soothe, to suppress, to invite, to pep up, to take off, to add on, to do almost anything. Sometimes, perhaps a good deal oftener than we in medicine would like to admit, this potent mixture of various medications interacting with each other, with the patient's own body chemistry, or with substances in the environment causes unexpected results, and things can go awry. Drugs can save our lives, but drugs can also kill.

It has been estimated that only about 10% of the drugs employed in the developed nations are administered to combat disease. A further disturbing estimate is that about 5% of all hospital admissions in the United States are because of deleterious drug effects. Iatrogenic disease—doctor-caused disease—is generally a result of drug toxicity, drug synergism, or allergy. Thus both

Drugs: The Good and the Bad

the medical profession and the public must be aware that modern medicines are not all blessing. Even though their good clearly outweighs their evil, they must be employed with caution and with restraint. The overuse of antibiotics is a case in point. These miracle drugs have saved countless lives, but because of their very effectiveness we have employed them far too widely and too indiscriminately. The result is that we are now seeing a significant increase in strains of bacteria resistant to them.

For example, the Center for Disease Control in Atlanta announced several years ago that at least one strain of gonorrhea had become resistant to penicillin, tetracycline, and ampicillin. Other serious diseases such as septicemia (blood poisoning), some types of pneumonia, malaria, and typhoid are not responding as they once did to treatment with the never-fail (hardly ever) antibiotics. This also helps explain the recent concern about the widespread employment of low-level doses of these drugs in animal feeds to promote growth. Research has suggested that this practice has greatly increased the pool of resistant bacteria. Hospitals have been reporting increasing incidences of resistant bacterial infections. Unfortunately, the resistant factor can be transferred from one bacterium to another nonresistant bacterium. This transfer occurs during conjugation, the process by which bacteria exchange nuclear material by forming a bridge between cells. The resistant factor (R-factor) is contained in that material, and in this rather simple manner the population of resistant bacteria increases.

Drugs can have undesirable effects on health in a number of ways. Toxicity occurs with overdosage of a medication usually and all too frequently in children who swallow potent drugs left carelessly within reach. An individual may even be poisoned by a normal dosage of a drug because of his or her own impaired metabolism or excretion; thus that person does not handle the drug as expected. Even exertion following some medications will hasten absorption through the medium of increased heart rate and blood flow. The result may be a toxic reaction.

Drugs may also have side effects. The *Physicians' Desk Reference* is loaded with horrifying possibilities, most of them remote for the majority of us. Some, however, can be serious, and the risks must be weighed against the benefits. Drugs may also have secondary effects. For example, a prolonged course of antibiotics may produce diarrhea when bacterial flora are altered and reduced.

Some people suffer from idiosyncratic reactions to certain drugs. They may have a reaction not unlike that of an allergic response but which does not have an immunological basis. This is thought to be a genetically produced abnormality. Prior exposure, such as is necessary for sensitization in allergy, is not required. Generally, the person who is idiosyncratic cannot tolerate even a very small amount of the drug. In this way idiosyncrasy differs from drug intolerance, for the intolerant individual may be able to tolerate some amount of the medication but not the normal amount.

One of the most serious problems drugs present is that of synergism, not only with another drug but, as we noted in the preceding chapter, with certain foods. A news item from London recently suggested some of the difficulties such syngerism can present. A gentleman suffering from hay fever inadvisedly washed down his allergy medications with an alcoholic beverage. After insulting passing motorists from a street-corner stance and upon relieving a policeman of his shirt, he found that a mixture of drugs and drink cost $50 in fines. In a more serious vein, drug interaction can be extremely hazardous. When, for example, a patient takes both tetracycline (an antibiotic) and phenothiazines (a psychotropic sedative), liver toxicity can result.

And then there is allergy to drugs. In the last decade or so physicians have become increasingly aware that some of modern medicine's most potent weapons against disease can trail sudden and unexpected consequences in their wake, the most frightening and life-threatening being an anaphylactic-shock reaction. Out of every 100 patients, two or three will develop an allergic reaction. Most such responses will be registered by the skin, and most will be mild, for although anaphylactic shock can occur, especially with drugs such as penicillin, drug reactions other than allergic are generally more hazardous. Nevertheless, physicians must keep the possibility of allergy in mind.

Allergy to drugs has a number of peculiarities. Some individuals may tolerate a drug, say, a medication such as aspirin, for weeks, months, even years, then suddenly suffer a severe allergic reaction to it. From that moment forward, even a minute exposure to the drug will produce symptoms. In addition, frequently a drug that is related pharmacologically will also produce allergy symptoms. Since a family history of allergy is not always present, it would appear that heredity is not a great factor in determining who develops drug hypersensitivity. In fact, it is believed that almost anyone could become allergic to certain drugs, given sufficient exposure. There are, however, several other factors which influence the chances of having an allergic reaction to a medication:

1. Route of administration of a drug. A drug applied to the skin or mucous membranes is the most likely to produce a reaction, whereas a drug

administered orally is least likely. A drug injected is somewhere in between. but when it does produce a reaction, it is frequently severe.

2. Amount and duration of exposure, with the added requirement of a particular interval between administrations of the drug.

3. General health of the individual. Patients who are debilitated or suffering from an infection appear to become sensitized more readily than essentially healthy patients.

4. Exposure and sensitization to a pharmacologically similar drug.

5. Whether the drug is contained in a medium and what that medium is. For example, penicillin administered in oil is more likely to produce a reaction than penicillin in water.

6. Condition of the skin at the site of administration. Medication applied to skin already injured increases the likelihood of sensitization.

7. Sex. More women suffer from drug allergy than do men. I am not at all sure why.

Another peculiarity of drug allergy is what is called a *fixed drug eruption* in which a drug causing a rash or lesions on some area of the body will produce the same symptoms on the same area when employed again. Drugs most often responsible for these repetitive symptoms are:

Amphetamines	Antihistamines
Barbiturates	Salicylates
Sulfonamides	Codeine

Some drugs frequently produce the same sequence of symptoms in various patients, although this is by no means a rigid rule. An example is aspirin, which more often than not produces hives and asthma among its allergic victims. Penicillin, which is feared for its penchant for producing anaphylactic shock, can often also produce an Arthus reaction (severe local inflammation at site of injection), drug fever, or, when applied to the skin, contact dermatitis. The sulfonamides leave their mark on the skin of patients with erythema multiforme (skin eruptions with dark red spots) or exfoliative dermatitis (chronic inflammation of the skin).

Drugs can also produce the strange symptom of photosensitivity, in which allergic patients are fine until they step out into the sunlight. When they do, they may turn beet red and itch like fury wherever their skin is exposed to the light. Even artificial light can cause this reaction for some hypersensitive people. The appearance of the skin may range from a sunburn-like condition to blisterlike lesions. Drugs most often responsible for this oddity are:

Phenothiazides   Sulfonamides

Tetracycline   Thiazine diuretics

Whereas some drugs are potent allergens in their own right, others have the ability to act as haptens, substances of low molecular weight which combine with proteins to sensitize. The hapten theory appears especially valid in drug allergy.

Whether a drug acts as an allergen alone or in combination, the results can be divided into three categories: an immediate reaction, an intermediate reaction, and a delayed reaction.

An immediate reaction occurs within minutes, even seconds of administration of the drug. It is characterized by such symptoms as hives, angioedema, rhinitis, asthma, gastrointestinal disturbances, conjunctivitis, Loeffler's syndrome (also called eosinophilic pneumonitis), and anaphylaxis. About one-third of the patients who suffer anaphylactic shock die.

An intermediate reaction occurs a day or so after a drug has been administered. Its symptoms may be similar to those of an immediate reaction, with the exception of anaphylaxis. Generally, symptoms also tend to be milder.

A delayed reaction, as could be expected, occurs days or even weeks following the administration of the drug and usually takes the form of dermatitis or of serum sickness. The former can be an Arthus type of reaction with rash, diffuse edema, hemorrhage, and ulcerative lesions. In other words, such a reaction can make a general mess of the patient. Serum sickness is characterized by fever, hives, joint pains, and arthritis. Lymphadenopathy (swollen, tender lymph glands), especially of the glands that drain the site of a drug injection, may also occur.

The patient with a history of allergy, especially of asthma and/or hives, tends to suffer an immediate drug reaction once sensitized, whereas the patient who has had no prior reaction to a medication and no particular history of allergy frequently suffers a delayed reaction once sensitized. I have noticed in my practice that although drug allergy appears somewhat different from other allergies, approximately one-third of the patients who suffer from hay fever also react to penicillin, often severely. I have also noticed that about one-third of my patients who are allergic to insect venom are also allergic to penicillin. What exactly are the relationships, if any, between these allergies, I have no idea.

If we examine a few of the drugs that cause allergic reactions we find that penicillin and aspirin head the list. Penicillin is a great medical discovery that has saved tens of thousands of lives, yet is perhaps one of the most common causes of severe drug reactions. It kills about 300 people each year and sends several thousand to the hospital. Some physicians believe the incidence of adverse reactions to it is rising, and it has been suggested that the practice of employing low-level amounts in animal husbandry has contributed to sensitizing more and more people to the antibiotic. Since penicillin used topically as in an ointment can also sensitize, many physicians prefer not to use it in this manner.

Symptoms of an immediate reaction to penicillin can range from local, such as a nodule at the injection site, to generalized, with widespread hives, angioedema, bronchospasm, and anaphylaxis. An intermediate reaction follows administration of the drug within two hours or up to two days and is usually characterized by hives and, sometimes, laryngeal edema. A delayed or serum-sickness type of reaction may appear anywhere from three days to two weeks following administration. Symptoms are usually hives, rash, fever, and arthralgia (joint pain).

To diagnose penicillin allergy the physician must rely heavily on the patient's history, for skin testing can be too dangerous with the possiblility of anaphylactic shock ever present. Penicillin disks are available for RAST testing, and this would be safe enough. Generally, however, there is little doubt about the matter, and once it is realized, the patient should make sure that he or she does not get the drug in the future. He or she should wear a medical warning tag or bracelet to alert any attending physician of this allergy, for it is possible that accident or illness could render him or her unconscious and unable to communicate. If there is a necessity for antibiotics to combat infection, erythromycin (which rarely produces allergy) or the tetracyclines can be administered.

One other antibiotic that can produce allergic reactions is neomycin. This drug is frequently employed in ointments and eye drops. In the former medication it can cause contact dermatitis and in the latter use, conjunctivitis.

I doubt that there is a medicine chest in the land that does not contain at least one bottle of aspirin in some form or other, buffered or unbuffered, combined with this or that other drug or simply plain. And allergy to aspirin is far more common than many people realize, perhaps simply because aspirin, acetylsalicylic acid, is an ingredient in so many over-the-counter nostrums that are touted for ailments that range from sniffles to headache, scratchy throat to aching joints. Exposure, therefore, is apt to be frequent and somewhat massive.

Allergic reactions to aspirin can be as severe as anaphylactic shock, although the most frequent responses are nasal congestion, asthma, hives, and angioedema. Less frequently, a reaction may manifest eczema or hemorrhage, with the latter probably due more to aspirin's irritant qualities than to allergy. Anyone allergic to aspirin should turn to the acetaminophen analgesics for relief from pain, Tylenol, for instance.

Insulin, the lifeline of the diabetic, may also cause allergic reactions, mainly with symptoms of hives and angioedema. Adults are the chief victims, for among juvenile diabetic patients on insulin for an extended period such reactions are rare. Why exactly is not known.

Reactions of one sort or another to blood transfusions are well known, but less than 50% of these are allergic in nature. Allergic symptoms generally manifested are chills and fever, rash, hives, and itching. Asthma is rare.

Finally, there are the vaccines and the toxoids. The needles and the new vaccination "guns" required for this rite of passage from birth to old age fill physicians' offices across the nation with the howls of immunized youngsters and expressions of dismay from their elders. Vaccines are cultured on a variety of mediums, chick embryos and animal (dog, rabbit, and the like) kidney cells for the most part. For a long time it was thought that anyone severely allergic to eggs should not receive vaccines prepared from chick embryo tissue, but this proposition is not universal. For example, children who are significantly hypersensitive to eggs seem to fare quite well with the measles vaccines cultured on chick embryo. Youngsters allergic to dog dander also apparently have little trouble with measles vaccine cultured on dog kidney cells.

German measles (rubella), however, presents a different picture. Generally cultured on duck embryo and dog or rabbit cells, these vaccines can produce an allergic response in anyone hypersensitive to feathers, fowl, or eggs, whereas those hypersensitive to animal dander may react to dog- or rabbit-cultured vaccines. For some reason, dog kidney cells seems especially allergenic for those allergic to dog dander, and such vaccine often produces a delayed reaction of some duration.

Vaccine for diphtheria, pertussis, and tetanus (DPT), which is the child's initial introduction to "the shots," rarely causes allergy problems. Tetanus toxoid, however, can cause serious reactions in older children and adults, especially the latter, producing symptoms which can include hives, generalized rash, localized edema, and that bugaboo of allergy, anaphylaxis.

Oral vaccines for poliomyelitis have caused no difficulties, but injected polio vaccines have resulted in some cases of allergic reaction, perhaps because of antibiotic traces incorporated in the vaccines.

Fortunately for many hypersensitive individuals, smallpox, that one-time scourge of humanity, has been wiped from the face of the earth. As far as I know at this writing, the only exceptions are some carefully guarded (it is to be hoped) strains left in several laboratories. Smallpox vaccination, which has literally left millions of tiny scars on the upper arms and thighs of generations, is no longer an automatic ordeal of childhood, nor is it even required for those who travel abroad. This is a happy state of affairs, for smallpox vaccination could trail some unpleasant consequences in its wake, and the vaccination itself is now considered far more of a risk than is any possibility of the disease being ressurected.

Other vaccines cultured on egg or chick embryo are more potent allergenically than the measles vaccine, although new techniques in producing vaccines and the use of less-potent antibiotics to prevent contamination, plus an increased use of avian tissue cultures, have reduced the problem significantly. We look more closely at this facet of allergy in a later chapter on the special problems of the allergic.

Diagnosis of allergy to drugs, as I mentioned, is based primarily on the patient's history. If the physician suspects a drug, other than aspirin or penicillin, and if there is no history of a prior reaction, he or she may challenge the patient with a small oral dose before prescribing normal doses or before injecting the medication. The physician will not attempt even this if there is a definite history of reaction. Thus anyone who has ever had an abnormal reaction to a drug should report it to the physician. Even if such a response was only a rash, the physician should know about it. In fact, once your skin has registered a reaction to a drug, it is more likely to do so to the same drug in the future and often more severely. This is especially true of topical applications of antibiotics.

Some people who are allergic to aspirin frequently are also allergic to foods containing salicylates. For a list of such foods see Appendix F.

GLOSSARY

Iatrogenic: doctor-caused disease or state of anxiety.

Conjugation: the process in which nuclear material is transferred between two bacteria or other specific life forms.

Idiosyncrasy: an exaggeration of the normal action of a drug.

Intolerance: an inability to tolerate normal dosages of a drug.

Arthus reaction: severe local inflammation at site of injection.

Photosensitivity: abnormal reaction of skin to sunlight (ultraviolet rays).

Erythema multiforme: skin eruption with dark red spots.

Exfoliative dermatitis: chronic scaly inflammation of the skin.

Lymphadenopathy: swollen and tender lymph glands; lymph-gland disease.

DPT: abbreviation for vaccine for diphtheria, pertussis (whooping cough), and tetanus.

SUMMARY

1. Adverse drug reactions account for an estimated 5% of hospital admissions in the United States.
2. Overusage of antibiotics has produced increasingly resistant bacteria.
3. Drugs cause health problems through various actions:

Toxicity

Side effects

Secondary effects

Idiosyncratic reactions

Intolerance reactions

Synergism

Allergic reactions

4. Drug allergy is generally registered by the skin with rashes, hives, angio-edema and eczema. However, anaphylactic shock can occur, especially with penicillin and aspirin.

5. Factors that play a role in drug allergy are:

Route of administration

Amount and duration of exposure

Presence of infection or general debilitation

Cross-reactivity

Medium employed with drug

Condition of site of administration

Sex

6. Individuals allergic to penicillin (or severely to any drug) should wear a medical warning tag or bracelet.

7. Allergic reactions to the culture medium of vaccines and toxoids or to the traces of antibiotics employed to prevent contamination are possible, though less likely than formerly.

8. Diagnosis of drug allergy depends primarily on the patient's history.

nine

*In memory of Timothy Ryan who died May 12th, 1814, in the 66th
year of his age.*

A thousand ways cut short our days
None are exempt from death.
A honey bee by stinging me
Did stop my mortal breath.
This grave contains the last remains
Of my frail house of clay.
My soul has gone not to return
To one eternal day.
Friends one and all both great and small
Behold where I do lie.
Whilst you are here for death prepare
Remember you must die.

Allergy to Insects

Dr. G.A. Dean reported this grim New England gravestone inscription in the *Journal of the American Medical Association* some years ago. Since it is so apropos to the discussion in this chapter, I have borrowed it. Even though Mr. Ryan's untimely end was long ago, it is still difficult for many people, physicians included, to believe that a tiny honeybee could cause the death of a healthy grown man. Yet, of course, this is the nature of allergy—it is not simply the instrument of reaction alone that causes the problem; rather, the degree of the individual's hypersensitivity in good part determines the magnitude of the response.

In any case, somewhere in the neighborhood of 40 to 100 such fatalities are reported each year in the United States. Many allergists, however, believe that these statistics represent only the tip of the iceberg, that many more deaths occur, which are reported as heart attacks or death by natural causes when in actuality they are due to swift and violent anaphylactic reactions to the injection of insect venom. One thing is certain, more people die in this country as a result of insect stings than they do from the bites of venomous snakes. Statistically, a honeybee is more dangerous than a rattlesnake.

Arthropoda (including insects) is a major division of the animal kingdom. In fact, its approximately 700,000 species make up over 80% of all animals on earth. Yet we scarcely notice their existence until they bite or sting us, make inroads in our gardens and crops, or become nuisances at picnics and the like. There they are, however, under our feet, in the air, on every bush and tree and flower; literally millions of large and small living things are going about the business of survival and of reproducing their kind. Someone possessed of infinite patience made a head count on 1 acre of land and came up with the figure of 425 million Arthropod inhabitants, which seems like an entirely respectable number of crawling, flying, slithering beings. I cannot vouch for this figure, having never attempted this kind of census taking, but it certainly is impressive. Those who propose that we turn to insects for nourishment to help keep food supplies abreast of growing human populations have an excellent suggestion. Insects are rich in protein, more so, it is said, than beef. We may well arrive at the day when the householder serves up termites fried in butter rather than call the exterminator.

In the meantime, there are the folks allergic to a good many members of these teeming insect populations. Whom should they fear? Table 9.1 describes those that cause the greatest difficulty for the hypersensitive, although let us quickly add that Arthropods can be helpful as well as harmful, and it behooves us to discriminate.

The chief stinging insects are among the ranks of Hymenoptera—the

Table 9.1: DESCRIPTION OF HARMFUL ARTHROPODS

Arthropod	Color and Shape	Food, Sound, Habits
Bumblebee	Burly, yellow and black	Loud drone
Honeybee	Brown-black	
Yellow jackets	Yellow, black stripes	Flowers, fruit
Sweat bees	Brown	
Hornets	Black, whitish markings	Fruit, aggressive
Fire ants	Bright red	Football-shaped nest
Mosquitoes	Delicate, varied color	High-pitched whine
Blackflies	Black-yellow, hump-backed	Persistent
Horseflies and deerflies	Black or black-white	
Stable flies	Brown-gray	
Sandflies	Brown, gray	
Biting midges	Black, tiny	Swarms
Wheel bugs	Coglike crest, mouse-gray	
Bedbugs	Red-brown	Leave black spots
Kissing bugs	Brown-black	
Puss caterpillar	Red-yellow hairs	
Buck moth	Pale green-gray	
Browntail	Brown-orange markings	
Fleas	Flat, dark brown	Jump
Head lice	Gray	Runs about head
Body lice	Creamy-white	On body and clothing
Pubic lice	Pink tinge	Inactive
Chiggers	Red	
Scabies	Gray-pink	Burrows
Scorpions	Black-yellow	
Black-widow spiders	Black-to-sepia with red hourglass marking	Coarse irregular web
	Shoe-button shape	
Brown recluse spider	Violin-shaped marking Brown-yellow	
Ticks	Baglike, brown, gray	

From *Parents' Guide to Allergy in Children,* Claude A. Frazier, M.D., Grosset & Dunlap, New York, 1978.

101

bees, hornets, wasps, and ants—and they are the most fascinating of all the Arthropods. They are also probably the most useful to man. Bees, for example, pollinate approximately one-third of our crops, especially citrus fruits and alfalfa. Without their efforts, orchards and hay fields would be unproductive. In fact, bees have become so valuable to agriculture that bee rustling has become a problem, with a ring of thieves that sneaks around the countryside, relieving farmers of their hives and selling them for premium prices.

We have long been entranced by the social orders of both honeybees and ants, and we have studied their communities tirelessly. Their ability to communicate with each other and their capacity for survival are awesome. It could be said that we have an affinity for their tiny hopes and woes, for we do not lump them in with the villainous, filthy, and pesky brand of insect such as flies and cockroaches. Even so, it is well to remember that any sting opens the way to infection and that this is a real possibility, especially after the sting of a yellow jacket or wasp, which are scavengers and likely to transmit bacteria with their venom.

The venom of Hymenoptera can cause either toxic reactions or allergic ones. A toxic reaction depends on the amount of venom injected through multiple stings and can range from the mild to the severe. It is estimated that 500 simultaneous stings or more can be fatal, and for some people fewer than this can cause death. Children may not survive more than 250 simultaneous stings. There are, however, cases on record of individuals surviving a good many more than these estimates. For instance, one physician has reported the case of a man who was attacked by a swarm of bees while walking along a riverbank in Africa. Even though he jumped into the water, plastered himself with mud and covered his head with his shorts, he received more than 2000 stings. He survived after spending five days in the hospital.

Symptoms of a toxic reaction resemble those of an allergic response with some minor differences. There is generally a greater incidence of gastrointestinal disturbances than in an allergic reaction, for instance, but other symptoms such as diarrhea, faintness, and unconsciousness are akin to those of an allergic response. Fever, drowsiness, headache, muscle spasm, and convulsions may also be present. Multiple stings may also produce hemoglobinuria, a condition in which hemoglobin is discharged in the urine as red blood cells disintegrate from the effects of the venom.

In contrast to a toxic reaction produced by multiple stings, an allergic reaction may be the product of a single sting. A single bee sting can be fatal for an extremely hypersensitive individual, for, as we have repeatedly noted, it is the individual's vulnerability that determines the extent of the reaction in the main.

A good deal of laboratory work has been done in recent years in an attempt to determine what substances in Hymenoptera venom are allergens and to what degree. Although a number of components have been sucessfully fractionated out of venom, there is still some uncertainty and some controversy as to their comparative potency. It has, however, been domonstrated that although the venoms of various members of Hymenoptera contain some similar substances and thus can cause the problem of cross-reactivity for many patients, they are not the same. Patients who react to only one of the stinging insects are reacting to a component specific to that species. If they react to several members of Hymenoptera, they are reacting to an allergen common to both. It is uncertain whether cross-reactivity is more common than venom specificity, for a good many patients have difficulty identifying their attacker, making it unclear whether the same insect is the offending agent or a different species has triggered the reaction.

Honeybees would leave human beings strictly alone, given their druthers. They are not inherently aggressive (with the so-called killer bees an outstanding exception), but people do tamper with their hives or disturb them among the flowers or step on them with bare feet or sandals while they are at work among the clover, and people do get stung. Honeybees can be especially irritable after a rain, since nectar and pollen may have been washed away, making it difficult for them to garner dinner. When it does sting, the honeybee stings but once, then goes off to die, its barbed stinger embedded in its victim, with venom sac and the bee's abdominal organs attached. That stinger, plus the still-pulsing venom sac, is the honey bee's calling card. It identifies the offending insect beyond a shadow of a doubt. Incidentally, the stinger and sac should be scraped out immediately with a knife or fingernail, for it is pumping more venom into the wound with each passing moment. It should never be squeezed with fingers or tweezers, since this simply forces more venom from the sac into the sting site.

Hornets, yellow jackets, and wasps do not possess barbed stingers; thus they can sting repeatedly, which, unfortunately, they tend to do. Yellow jackets have frequent victims, both because they are unusually aggressive and because they often build their nests in ground holes or at the base of posts and poles. People are apt to step in the former and knock against the latter, and in either case, yellow jackets swarm to the attack. They are not only speedy flyers, they also follow their victim for some distance, making escape difficult. Hornets, too, can be encountered by the unwary, since they frequently hang their football-sized papier-mâché nests in bushes, hedges, or from low-hanging tree limbs. A little prior research into such places would go a long way toward preventing unexpected meetings.

Wasps often haunt the homes of human beings. They not only build their paperlike nests under eaves and windowsills, but when cold weather sets in, they boldly invade the house itself in a search for shelter. Many a victim of their wrath came on them nestled in a pair of pants, a folded shirt, or a blanket.

The fire ant and the harvester ant are the villains among the ant world, with the former the greater menace, perhaps simply because of its massive invasion of the South. The imported fire ant, brought to this country accidentally from South America, has become a real problem in thirteen Southern states. Its venom not only differs from that of other Hymenoptera, but also from that of other ant species. Its manner of stinging is also unique. It seizes its victims with its mandibles, and once it has attained a bulldog grip, it pivots, using the stinger on its rear end to inflict a number of fiery lesions. Fiercely aggressive when its nest is disturbed, fire ants will pour out by the thousands and within seconds swarm over the clumsy foot that has come too close or the unfortunate animal that has blundered into the mound. It has been reported that fire ants have killed pigs, chickens, quail, and even new-born calves dropped by the cow too close to fire-ant mounds. Fire ants also will invade the home in search of food and thus come into contact with unwary human beings.

Reactions to Hymenoptera venom can be classified as follows:

Toxic, which we have already discussed

Normal

Local

Immediate generalized systemic (allergic)

Delayed, like serum sickness

Psychological

Those who suffer a normal reaction to Hymenoptera stings generally feel a sharp pain at the sting site, then exhibit a bit of redness, perhaps a little swelling, and often subsequent itching. Usually, that's all there is to it, although the victim should give the sting area a thorough washing with soap and water to ensure against the possibility of secondary infection. An ice pack or a paste of baking soda and water will help take the pain from the event.

A local reaction goes a bit further than this by producing significant swelling in the area of the sting, generally classified as edema covering more than a 2-inch diameter around the site. When such edema covers two or more body joints, it is wise to consult a physician, for such a significant degree of swelling may presage an allergic reaction on the next encounter with the insect. Also, if such swelling seems larger each time one is stung, this, too, may signal the possibility of a hypersensitive reaction in the future.

An allergic or generalized systemic reaction differs entirely from normal and local reactions, because it is not confined to the sting site, but rather is registered by other body systems, including the respiratory system, the cardiovascular system, and the skin. Such a reaction can range from the mild to the almost instantly fatal. It has been estimated that between 1 and 2 million Americans are at risk of suffering a severe allergic response to Hymenoptera venom.

Initial symptoms of an allergic reaction may begin mildly enough, with itching around the eyes and mouth, a slight cough, flushing, and a feeling of overall warmth. Matters may stop here, but unfortunately, not for everyone. Symptoms may intensify rapidly, with widespread hives, constriction of throat and chest, nausea and vomiting, breathing difficulties, weakness, falling blood pressure, cyanosis, collapse, loss of consciousness, and death.

Such a reaction may appear to have arrived out of the blue to puzzle both patient and physician. Often patients will insist that they have been stung many times before with no more than normal reactions, or they may state that they have never been stung and so could not have been sensitized. It takes prior exposure, the reader will remember, to set one up for an allergic response. In the first incidence, prior stings with their normal reactions did sensitize patients and put their IgE antibodies too insistently on guard. In the second incidence they may simply have forgotten childhood encounters with Hymenoptera, for it is possible for sensitization to have taken place years prior to an allergic response, and those initial symptoms of a normal reaction may have been so mild that little was made of it. IgE antibodies have an unhappy faculty of being able to persist for years after a single sting, although in many individuals there is apparently a rise in IgE production immediately following the sting, then a gradual fall, with a corresponding rise in IgG-blocking antibodies. There is, however, a good deal still to be learned about this process.

Location of the sting may also affect the severity of the symptoms.

A sting in the head or neck region is apt to be serious, since the subsequent edema in this area can obstruct the victim's airway. A sting in close proximity to the eye, especially a sting on the eyelid, may injure the eye itself. A severe generalized systemic reaction can intensify into anaphylactic shock within minutes of a sting. Fatal outcomes frequently occur within the first 10 to 15 minutes following a sting and sometimes within 3 to 5 minutes. It is generally thought that if the victim survives the first half hour, he or she will be all right. Because symptoms of anaphylaxis are similar to those of heart attack and because sting wounds themselves are tiny and often obscured by hair or clothing, misdiagnosis may be fairly frequent. As an example, not long ago a well-known journalist was stung while jogging. Even though he told a companion that he had been stung and even though the autopsy report indicated that anaphylaxis occurred, death was attributed to heart trouble. And because misdiagnosis can lead to delayed or wrong treatment, it is very important that anyone who has had an allergic reaction to insects wear a medical warning tag or bracelet.

Determining which member of Hymenoptera is responsible for an allergic reaction can present a problem for the physician, because many patients cannot tell one stinger from another even if fortunate enough to see the attacker. The honeybee, as we have noted, leaves its calling card and is no problem, but generally, in their haste to put some distance between themsilves and the attackers, most patients cannot even describe their assailants. Where the attack occurred and what the patient was doing at the time can be helpful in identification. Skin tests may help, but they are not totally reliable. Nor is the newer RAST technique.

Is it important to identify the offending insect?

It is to be preferred, but in the past when hyposensitization therapy was administered using whole-body extracts, it was possible to use mixed Hymenoptera extracts to protect against several suspected species. Now that venom extracts are being employed, it may be much more important to be able to identify the insect involved. The great hope, I believe, is that someday in the near future we will be able to extract only those substances in venom which cause allergic reactions and even, perhaps, to find a way to synthesize such substances.

Hyposensitization (or desensitization as it is also called) is the process of injecting extracts of allergenic substances in ever-increasing strengths and at set intervals, until patients reach a level at which they can tolerate a normal exposure to the allergen. For example, if the physician finds a barbed stinger in a patient's wound after an encounter with a member of the Hymenoptera clan, the physician will begin hyposensitization with whole-body honeybee extracts or the new honeybee venom extracts. The injections will be gradually increased in strength until the patient can tolerate at least several stings without symptoms of an allergic reaction. Once at this level of tolerance, the patient receives a periodic maintenance injection. Allergists used to think that after three years the patient would arrive at permanent tolerance, but after a number of patients slipped back into hypersensitivity after this period, allergists began to recommend 10 years of maintenance to ensure protection. However, we are not certain that 10 years does provide adequate protection. Many allergists are now saying that maintenance should be indefinite until research indicates when and if permanent tolerance is reached.

Although venom extracts are being newly employed on a wide clinical basis in hyposensitization, they have been around for many years. Dr. Mary Lovelace pioneered their development, but the difficulty of extraction was a stumbling block. Removing Hymenoptera venom from tiny venom sacs was no easy task. So whole-body extracts in which the bodies of the insects were crushed, venom sacs and all, have been employed for many years, very successfully, in my opinion. Nor am I alone in this belief, for a number of my colleagues believe that WBE, as whole-body extracts are called, has protected most of the patients receiving hyposensitization therapy. However, recent research has suggested that venom extracts are far more protective, although they have not yet been employed on a clinical basis of any magnitude. There is also some concern whether these potent extracts can be used with safety in a general clinical setting for a cross section of patients.

The process of venom extraction from honeybees is interesting and reasonably sinple. Worker bees are placed on a plastic membrane and given enough of an electric shock to make them sting through the membrane, but not to kill them. Since the membrane is thin, they can withdraw their stingers without harm and live to sting again. In the meantime, the venom has been collected beneath the membrane and started on its way through the process of producing extracts. Wasps and hornets do not fare as well. They are frozen, and their venom sacs are dissected under microscopes and punctured to let the venom escape. Then the result is buffered to separate the remaining body proteins of the sacs. As can be imagined, this procedure is difficult and expensive.

Since nothing in medicine is 100% certain, patients being hyposensitized should keep an insect-sting kit handy. In fact, it is my recommendation that even after a maintenance dosage is reached, anyone allergic to insect stings should possess three such kits and keep one in the home, one in the car, and one on the person whenever and wherever Hymenoptera could be encountered. These kits, available only on a physician's prescription, contain a premeasured dose of epinephrine (adrenalin), the one drug capable of halting anaphylactic shock in its tracks long enough for the victim to get to medical help. Probably the simplest type of kit for the nonmedical patient is the kind that contains a preloaded sterile syringe of premeasured adrenalin. All the kits contain a tourniquet, sealed alcohol pads, and simple, clear instructions. Even when mild symptoms of an allergic reaction follow a sting, it is wise to employ the adrenalin at once, for anaphylactic shock has a nasty way of intensifying so rapidly that loss of consciousness within minutes is a good possibility. The adrenalin is injected just beneath the skin of the outer upper arm or the upper thigh just above the knee. The latter is the easiest spot for self-administration.

It is important to note that the adrenalin is a stop-gap only and that the victim must be gotten to the nearest hospital or physician's office as quickly as possible for further necessary treatment. The kit is designed to abate rapidly intensifying symptoms of a severe, generalized, systemic reaction long enough to accomplish just this, for many victims of insect stings find themselves far from medical aid. The adrenalin furnishes life-saving time.

I always recommend to my insect-allergic patients that they, like those allergic to foods and drugs, wear a medical warning tag or bracelet. I also provide my patients with a list of do's and don't's to help avoid stinging insects as much as is humanly possible, for there is no use in deliberately courting fate, no matter how well protected one is. This list can be found in Appendix G.

Before leaving Hymenoptera, we must consider ants briefly, especially fire ants. Although allergic reactions to ant stings are similar to allergic reactions to their Hymenoptera cousins, normal reactions are quite different. Most normal reactions to ant stings other than the fire ant are mildly painful and perhaps will itch a little. Fire-ant stings are something else again. They are extremely painful, which is where the word *fire* comes in, for it is completely descriptive of the kind of pain this small but fiercely aggressive creature can inflict. Fire-ant venom is necrotic but, oddly enough, has an antibiotic quality which causes the pus-filled lesions it creates to be sterile. These pustules persist for several days, often a week or more. Sometimes haloed in red, they soon form a crust and scar tissue. On occasion the damage to tissue can be so great as to require skin grafting. Diagnosis is simple, not only because of the unusual appearance of the lesions but also because they form a circular pattern, the hallmark of the fire ant, which, as we noted earlier, bites with its mandibles, then pivots, stinging all the way.

Hyposensitization with whole-body extracts of fire ants has proved exceedingly effective in protecting patients allergic to their venom. Unfortunately, so far there is no way to protect against normal reactions to their venom other than complete avoidance of these savage little ants.

Allergy to insect bites tends to be far less severe than it is to insect stings and, except for several members of Arachnida (spiders, scorpions, and the like), toxic reactions are rare. The allergens involved in hypersensitivity reactions are generally in the saliva that the insect injects into a wound when it bites, often to soften or liquify tissues to make it easier to suck up dinner. Actually, these substances sometimes predigest the meal before the insect takes a mouthful.

Biting insects which commonly cause allergy are mosquitoes, deerflies, blackflies, horseflies, fleas, scabies, lice, and kissing bugs. As we have noted, many insects can also be the cause of allergy if inhaled or ingested.

Mosquitoes are ubiquitous. As many a schoolchild knows, they are infamous transmitters of disease, causing health problems ranging from malaria to encephalitis. The female is the bloodthirsty sex who has now and again directed the affairs of humanity. An excellent example is the exchange of the Panama Canal project from a French engineering feat to an American medical success story. In order to perpetuate the mosquito population, the female must have blood, whereas the male, a Mr. Milquetoast of the insect world, is perfectly content with plant juices and nectar. When she sucks the blood of an individual suffering from a disease, then goes off to dine on a healthy person, she is very likely to present the latter with whatever it is the former is suffering from, carried within the saliva she injects.

Mosquitoes have dining preferences. The ladies will not take their meals from just anyone. Experiments have indicated that some people have built-in repellents in their skin lipids (fat). It has also been demonstrated that to sweat is to issue a clear invitation to mosquitoes to come to dinner. They also prefer a sweating person to be puffing a good bit of carbon dioxide into the air—someone who is exercising strenuously or has just been doing so. They have a penchant for dark colors, dark skin, and estrogen, too. The latter is especially present during a woman's menstrual cycle; thus an olive-skinned woman wearing navy blue, playing tennis, inclined to perspire freely, and into her monthly period is a prime mosquito target unless she possesses lipids that repel.

A mosquito's bite generally leaves a red wheal and causes deplorable itching. Although the biting mechanism of the mosquito at work on our hide causes some of our discomfort, the lion's share is the result of allergenic substances in its saliva. There are two types of reaction to that saliva: an immediate one with wheal and itch and a delayed reaction occurring hours later with a pimplelike lesion, often accompanied by some swelling and a good deal of even more intense itching. Experimenters have demonstrated the role of saliva in all this by cutting the salivary ducts of a mosquito, then letting it bite a victim. When the ducts were severed, no symptoms resulted from the bite.

Other experiments have demonstrated that many individuals eventually arrive at a stage in which they enjoy relative immunity from symptoms caused by a mosquito bite, but only after suffering repeated attacks.

Severe allergic reactions to mosquito bites are rare, and although there are cases in the literature detailing such severe responses, I have never heard of a fatality. Secondary infections as a result of inordinate scratching are anything but rare. Thus the first step in the treatment of mosquito bites is to wash the bite areas thoroughly with soap and water. An oral antihistamine is helpful in relieving the mighty itch. Hyposensitization to mosquito bites has been fairly effective, although nowhere nearly as effective as it has been for Hymenoptera stings. Still, anyone who has suffered severe reactions and a good deal of discomfort should consider giving it a try. It is well worth the effort, especially for those who respond to the onslaught of mosquitoes with nausea, generalized hives, and dizziness.

Biting flies are as much of a summertime nuisance as female mosquitoes and far more likely to produce severe allergic reactions. Deerflies, blackflies, horseflies, and biting midges are the most allergenically potent and are capable of causing anaphylactic responses in those who are especially hypersensitive. In addition, their bites are apt to be quite painful, especially those of horseflies and deerflies. Although horseflies bite hard, they tend to bring less-severe reactions than their smaller deerfly cousins, perhaps because they are large and noisy, thus giving the victim a chance to squash them before the damage is great. The deerfly, on the other hand, not only inflicts a good deal of pain but is also responsible for some especially severe reactions—evidently some strange ones as well. For example, a colleague wrote me about a girl who was bitten under her big toe with such marked subsequent swelling of the foot that walking became difficult. My correspondent wrote that the only treatment the girl received was an old folk remedy that entailed sticking the infected part into lake sand. Apparently it worked, although I haven't the faintest idea why.

Deerflies and horseflies are also transmitters of disease, such as tularemia and anthrax.

Blackflies are as vicious as deerflies and far more numerous. They literally swarm about their victim on occasion and have been known to send large animals stampeding into lakes and rivers to escape their bites. Since blackfly bites often raise considerable swelling, it is thought that there could be a toxic element in their saliva. In any case, they draw blood as well as curses, and some individuals become highly sensitive to their bites. One school of thought believes that, as in the case of mosquitoes, people develop a natural immunity after repeated bites and can tolerate the blackflies quite well. However, another theory explains such decreases in the intensity of reactions as a decrease in the potency of blackfly toxins which may be seasonal in their production, being highly potent at one time, far less at another.

Like mosquitoes, blackflies appear to exercise some degree of preference in their choice of victims. They are more attentive to those who wear bright colors and exude a goodly amount of carbon dioxide.

Biting midges can be almost as much of a pest as blackflies and can inflict almost as much discomfort. They swarm to the attack, usually at dawn and/or dusk, but on gray, cloudy days they may be ready to dine any time of day. Their bites are painful and can raise welts the size of mosquito bites, which makes it fortunate that they are no bigger. If they were as large as a mosquito, their bite might be worse than the horsefly's. Because of the intense itching they produce, scratching is almost unavoidable; thus secondary infection is a good probability. As with fly bites of any kind, washing with soap and water is the best of all ways to prevent such complications, and oral antihistamines are helpful in reducing the urge to scratch.

Hyposensitization to fly bites has not been totally successful for all persons and all varieties of the biting flies, but, again, for the severely allergic, such therapy is well worth a try. Hyposensitization to deerflies has been particularly effective and should be undertaken by anyone who reacts with severe symptoms.

Kissing bugs belong to the family Reduviidae, which are often called assassin bugs, because of their predilection for dining on soft-bodied insects. The kissing bug got its amorous name because of its habit of biting its victims on the face as they sleep. They dine on blood and can be an instrument both to transmit disease and to produce an allergic reaction. Their bites are usually painless, and their victims wake up in the morning somewhat surprised to find that they have been attacked. There are a number of cases on record of severe allergic reactions to their bites, including anaphylactic shock. Several years ago a California man succumbed after repeated bites had intensified his sensitivity. Even though he had possessed an insect-sting kit and had to administer the adrenalin in prior reactions, his final encounter with a kissing bug evidently resulted in loss of consciousness and death before he could help himself. Hyposensitization to kissing bugs has been quite effective and should be administered to anyone who has had generalized systemic symptoms.

Fleas, chiggers, bedbugs, scabies mites, and other insects may cause allergic reactions. Fleas cause an eruption often called papular urticaria. Somewhat hivelike wheals ranging in color from bright red to brown are generally grouped on arms and legs, face and neck, or shoulder and hip areas, wherever, in fact, clothing is apt to be snug. They itch. As with mosquito bites, people seem to develop an immunity against flea-bite reactions after a good bit of exposure. For example, newcomers to California complain loudly and bitterly about something that bites, whereas oldtimers scarcely notice that their state is overrun with fleas.

Treatment of flea bites, like all insect bites, begins with washing the area carefully with soap and water. Antihistamine and antipruritic drugs (Temaril) help relieve the almighty itch. Flea powdering one's pets regularly, with special attention to their bedding or favorite curling-up corners, will help keep flea populations in check. Hyposensitization to fleas has not been effective and may even enhance the patient's sensitivity.

Chiggers, like the house-dust mite, are members of the order Acarina and parasites on all of us animals with a backbone. They must have a blood meal to advance themselves from the larval stage, and so they hang around in the bushes or on tall stalks of grass and wait for an unwary dinner of blood to come along. They aren't the least choosy, for birds and snakes as well as furry animals and human beings will do. When it bites, the chigger secretes a substance that liquifies the skin cells so that the chigger can suck up the result. Long after the chigger has dropped off, the saliva substance continues to irritate the site and to create the awful itch that is characteristic of a chigger attack. Secondary infection, therefore, is a very real possibility. Starch baths before bedtime and the application of calamine lotion to the bite areas offer relief, and oral antihistamines may also be helpful. Some people are far more sensitive to chigger invasion than others and on occasion may even need a sedative to relieve their discomfort.

The scabies mite is exceedingly prevalent across the land at this writing. In fact, its presence has been cited as an epidemic, for the scabies-mite population waxes and wanes in a regular cycle, even in the most modern of nations. The female scabies mite burrows into the skin to lay its eggs at the end of the tunnel. Initially, the victim may be unaware of its presence, but after a few weeks or a month, that presence becomes known in the form of itching, fierce itching, caused, it is believed, by the various toxins it releases. Vesicles and redness appear in the areas of the burrows, and, because of that itch, secondary infection can occur. Treatment is usually an application of a scabicide such as gamma benzene hexachloride following a warm bath with the liberal use of soap. One application over the entire body from the neck down is usually sufficient. A 5% sulfur ointment or a 10% strength can be substituted, but it is somewhat smelly and messy. In any case, following treatment all clothing and bedding for the entire family should be laundered. Calamine lotion and sedatives may still be necessary after the scabies mite has been disposed of, since itching is likely to continue some time after it is gone.

Although most of us in the United States associate bedbugs with run-down hotels and "flea bags," the great majority of people on earth live cheek by jowl with these tiny, reddish-brown, flat-bodied creatures. Bedbugs bite, but since they usually bite at night and since they evidently inject an anesthetic substance, the victims generally are unaware that they have been under attack until they wake the next morning to find the reddish wheals in a linear pattern of one, two, three on their skin. Some individuals are highly sensitive to the bedbug and may exhibit significant swelling and even generalized symptoms, including anaphylaxis. Treatment consists of relieving discomfort and itching with starch baths and calamine lotion, with oral antihistamines as needed. Secondary infection should be guarded against.

Spiders also may produce allergic reactions in hypersensitive individuals, but their main hazard is toxic. Two species in the United States, the black widow and the brown recluse, can inflict severe, even fatal reactions. Several species of scorpions in the Southwest are also very poisonous. In general, however, the insects covered in this chapter are responsible for most of the allergic responses physicians see. Avoidance and preventive measures for those who respond uncomfortably to their attentions can be found in Appendix G.

GLOSSARY

Arthropoda: a division of the animal kingdom that includes the classes of Insecta and of Arachnida.

Hymenoptera: membrane-winged; an order of insects that includes bees, hornets, wasps, yellow jackets, and ants.

Acarina: the order of Arachnids that includes mites.

Lipids: fats and fatlike substances insoluble in water.

Estrogen: female sex hormone produced by ovarian follicle.

Necrotic: capable of causing death of tissue.

SUMMARY

1. Arthropods make up over 80% of the animal kingdom.

2. Insects that cause the most common health problems for persons in the United States are bees, hornets, wasps, ants, flies, mosquitoes, scabies mites, chiggers, fleas, and bedbugs.

3. Insect bites and stings can cause either toxic or allergic reactions, and sometimes both.

4. In the wound honeybees leave barbed stingers, which should always be scraped out, never squeezed.

5. Wasps, hornets, and yellow jackets are scavengers capable of transmitting pathogens with their venom.

6. Fire-ant venom differs from that of other members of Hymenoptera and is necrotic in action.

7. Even mild systemic reactions to insect stings or bites should receive medical attention as quickly as possible.

8. Injectable adrenalin is the only drug capable of abating intensifying symptoms of anaphylactic shock.

9. Stings in the neck and eye region can have serious consequences, such as obstruction of the airways due to edema and injury to the eye itself.

10. Hyposensitization for allergic reactions to insect stings is effective but is less successful for allergy to most insect bites.

11. Although not a new technique, insect-venom extracts are now available for the first time for clinical use.

12. Anyone allergic to insect stings or bites should keep an insect-sting kit handy, should wear a medical warning tag or bracelet, and should practice the avoidance and preventive measures listed in Appendix G.

ten

We have dealt with allergens inhaled, ingested, and injected, so now it is time to consider allergens contacted—those substances we encounter with our skin, frequently to the detriment of the perfection of our appearance. Our skin is a marvelous protective envelope in which we arrive into the world stamped and sealed. But it is also a vulnerable envelope, since it must meet that world head on—well, at least, out in front. And there are a number of things out there capable of marring the human hide, especially the hide of the allergic simply because they have a greater penchant than the rest of us for erupting in lesions, rashes, hives, eczema, oozes, and crusts. We add the word *contact* to these various manifestations of dermatitis to distinguish the kind of skin problems caused by contacting allergens rather than those caused by allergens (or other things) ingested or inhaled or injected.

Contact dermatitis is not always a product of allergy, however. It can be caused by irritation of the skin by harsh chemicals or plants in which no immunological factor is involved. What we deal with in this chapter is allergic contact dermatitis, with hypersensitivity to various substances at the root of the problem.

Do Not Touch: Allergic Contact Dermatitis

When we are very young we are constantly being exhorted not to touch. This is excellent advice for those who suffer from contact allergy, and it may be a lifelong admonition, for some allergens are so potent and some people's hypersensitivity so strong that the skin reacts messily and, in some cases, the mucous membranes also to contact with the allergenic substance. Poison ivy is a good example of both allergenic potency and individual sensitivity. It is so potent that its ability to mar the human hide is all but universal. It is a rare person who does not come out the worse for wear after contact with the shiny "leaves of three." There are some people, however, who end up in the hospital after such an encounter, so exquisite is their sensitivity.

Contact dermatitis can be mild or severe, immediate or delayed, chronic or acute. Symptoms can range from a few lesions or a mild rash to weeping, crusting vesicles that cover wide areas of the skin. As with other aspects of allergy, contact dermatitis depends on a number of factors for its existence and its severity. The degree of the individual's hypersensitivity and the potency of the allergen involved are foremost, with duration and intensity of exposure following close behind. Irritation of the skin or the presence of infection can also be important factors.

Contact allergens can be met just about anywhere in the environment—in plants, foods, metals, drugs, cosmetics, clothing, and detergents and chemicals, both those in industrial and household use, not to mention out on the farm.

Contact dermatitis is no respecter of age. The very young may exhibit it in the form of diaper rash, with the sensitizing agent the detergent used to wash the nappies. Or the baby may respond to the pleasant-smelling, soothing lotion applied to urine-irritated skin. In one bizarre case, an infant broke out in dermatitis in a perfect imprint of its mother's lips when she kissed the infant just after having dined on eggs. The baby was acutely sensitive to eggs, as the reader might guess. In another somewhat odd case, a gentleman made a present of a mink coat to his lady fair. Unfortunately, she did not remain beautiful for long, for she turned out to be allergic to mink (imagine!) and broke out in a fancy dermatitis.

In the middle years occupational contact dermatitis plays a large role in skin problems, and in advancing age topical drugs often are a factor. From birth until death individuals whose skin registers their hypersensitivities will come into contact with any number of things capable of producing dermatitis.

To return to that potent contactant, poison ivy, this plant and its cousins of the Rhus family—poison oak and poison sumac—contain a sensitizing agent, called urushiol or pentadecycatechol, in the oleoresins of the saps. This agent is almost completely nonvolatile and thus can be carried about on just about anything it comes in contact with—clothing, animal fur, or tools. Those who think to get rid of the Rhus plants by burning must do so with caution, since breathing the smoke may affect the respiratory system. On the plant itself, the sap is in the leaves, stem, bark, and roots, but the pollen at least is free of allergenic substances. Poison ivy is so potent that it is said that if you wore a coat that contacted the plant, hung the coat in a closet, then took it down a year later, you could come down with a case of poison ivy wherever your skin contacted the contaminated area of the coat.

Hyposensitization to poison ivy and poison oak is controversial, with success claimed by some and failure admitted by others. One thing is certain: such therapy should not be initiated during the active phase of the allergy, for it could not only make matters worse as far as the dermatitis is concerned, it could also result in kidney damage.

Avoiding Rhus is the best of all preventive measures and "leaves of three, turn and flee" should be learned early in life.

Other plants can cause dermatitis on contact, although they are neither as potent nor as ubiquitous as the Rhus family. Some individuals who suffer hay fever in response to inhaled ragweed may find themselves responding to contact with the pollen with dermatitis as well. Some of the handsomest of plants can make contact unforgettable. Geraniums, for example, that brighten a window may also brighten the skin of the hypersensitive. Chrysanthemums and philodendron can produce a dermatitis that is similar to that of poison ivy. The pollen of the former may float about to produce a rash on contact, especially on the eyelids, since the skin of the lids is especially tender and vulnerable. Florists and professional gardeners commonly suffer such rashes.

The substances in plant tissues which sensitize range from the phenols in poison ivy to the terpenes in the peel of citrus fruits. The latter is also contained in turpentine obtained from pine trees and is the factor that can cause havoc on the hands of an allergic painter who uses turpentine to clean up after a job. Youngsters who play among the buttercups and try to see who likes butter by holding the bright yellow flowers under each others' chins may turn up with that odd offshoot of allergy, photosensitivity. The area of the skin that has contacted the plant, then been exposed to the sun, can turn up with a bright red rash. Mustard, celery, and carrots can also produce this startling effect. And gardeners should be aware that when they weed among tomato plants, eggplants, and potato rows, they run the risk of severe dermatitis either from allergy or from irritant substances contained in these plants. Children love to roll down a hillside, and the longer and thicker the grass, the softer the tumble. Some children, however, go home with a rash.

Contact dermatitis to metals is fairly common, and nickel heads the list

Table 10.1: TABLE OF CONTACTANTS AND THEIR SOURCES

Contactant	Source	Distribution of Lesions	Comments
Aluminum Chlorhydroxide	Deodorants, antiperspirants	Axillae	
Aniline	Dyes, drugs, inks, paints	Exposed areas and areas of perspiration	
Bergamot	Shalimar perfume, toilet water	Neck, etc.	Photosensitizer
Bithionol	Soaps, shampoos, cosmetics	Exposed areas	
Carmine	Lipsticks, rouges	Lips, face, eyelids	
Cement	Occupational	Exposed areas, inside feet	Use open patch test
Chlorobenzene	Insecticides	Face, neck	
Cobalt chloride	Cement, hair dyes, pigments, pottery	Exposed areas	Acneiform
Copper sulfate	Insecticides, coins, fertilizers	Exposed areas	Rare
DDT	Insecticides	Exposed areas	
Formalin (40% solution of formaldehyde gas)	Antiperspirants, nail hardener, permanent wave lotions	Depends on source	
	Insecticides, embalming fluid, perma-pressed clothes, paper, photography		
Hexachlorophene	Soaps, antiperspirants, topical dermatologicals, shampoos	Depends on source	
Lanolin	Cosmetics, pharmaceuticals	Depends on source	
Mercaptobenzothiazole	Shoes, rubber objects	Depends on source	
Neomycin	Topical medications, cosmetics, soaps	Depends on source	

Contactant	Source	Distribution of Lesions	Comments
Nickel sulfate	Zippers, jewelry, snaps, buttons, metal chairs, door handles, eyeglass frames, bobby pins, cookware, tools, umbrellas, nickel-containing alloys, nickel-plating, needles, pins, scissors, handbags, belt buckles, wiring, fungicides, insecticides, medical and dental instruments	Local and may simulate atopic dermatitis	Common
Paraphenylenediamine	Hair dyes, leather processing, printer's ink, lithography, X-ray fluids	Areas of increased perspiration	Common
Pentadecylcatechol	Rhus family of plants	Exposed areas mostly	Common, streaks
Potassium Dichromate	Leather, matches, yellow paint, detergents, cement, rubber	Shoe dermatitis	
Tetrachlorosalicylanilide	Soaps	Exposed areas	Photosensitizer
Tetramethylthiuram disulfide	Rubber	Feet (shoes)	
Tribrominatedsalicylanilide	Soaps	Exposed areas	Photosensitizer
Turpentine	Polishes, varnishes, solvents, insecticides, liniments, ointments	Depends on source	Cross-reacts with ragweed and chrysanthemum

Melvin L. Elson, M.D. in *Current Therapy of Allergy*, 2nd ed., Claude A. Frazier, M.D., Ed., Medical Examination Publishing, Garden City, N.Y., 1978, pp. 90–92.

of offending agents, perhaps because it is so widely employed in a variety of objects worn next to the skin, such as zippers and watchbands, or frequently handled, such as coins and keys. Unfortunately, when nickel contacts sweaty skin, the chloride in the sweat releases nickel salts. Those salts are potent sensitizers, especially if there is additional mechanical irritation. The extent of the resulting dermatitis depends on whether the nickel is contained in an alloy and what that alloy is. Sometimes an alloy of two metals is a more potent sensitizer than each of the metals alone; on the other hand, sometimes metals that sensitize in their own right tend to cancel each other out when combined.

Workers who handle nickel frequently suffer an itching rash on their hands, but oddly enough, the rash may migrate from the site of actual contact to other areas of the body. This strange characteristic makes diagnosis of nickel dermatitis somewhat difficult. Generally, however, contact with nickel sets its mark plainly on the skin—on the wrist where a watch is worn, on the earlobes where earrings dangle, on the neck where chains and necklaces adorn, on odd places of the body where zippers and skin have met. Not too many years ago nickel garter fasteners set their imprint on the upper thighs of girdle-wearing ladies, but these days I venture that few physicians see these signs of fashion—and of constraint.

Among bartenders, waiters, barbers, bank clerks, and even members of the medical profession, constant contact with nickel in "silverware," scissors, coins, and medical instruments produces considerable dermatitis. Strangely, cement workers and housewives are also often among nickel's victims, the former because of the nickel traces in cement and the latter because such traces are also often in household detergents.

Chromium is probably the next most frequent cause of metal sensitization, in fact, there is often cross-reactivity between nickel and chromium. Cobalt also cross-reacts with these two metals, although most of us do not come into contact with it frequently. Chromium dermatitis can be an occupational problem in industries ranging from the manufacture of automobiles to photographic supplies. The dermatitis it produces is often ulcerous in nature, and because chromium compounds are frequently soluble in both water and body fluids, the problem tends to spread.

Although other metals may produce contact dermatitis, they are not as potent as nickel, chromium, and cobalt. Mercury gave a good deal of trouble in the past when it was widely employed in ointments and topical medications of various kinds. It can still cause a problem when thermometers break or electric batteries are contacted or burned, and once in a great while someone turns up allergic to the mercury amalgam used to fill a cavity in a tooth.

As we have noted in the earlier chapter on drug allergy, one of the side effects of our ever-increasing pharmacopeia, with its annual introduction of new medications, has been the sensitization of a good many people. Topical

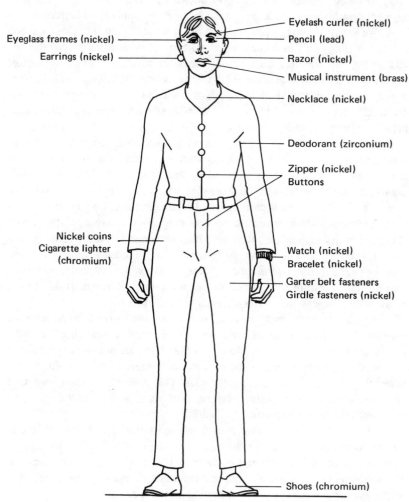

Metal dermatitis can turn up in some unlikely places on the human body.

mercury medications aren't the only ones to make matters worse on occasion. Neomycin, for example, is quick to cause contact dermatitis in the hypersensitive. Fortunately, other antibiotics which rarely cause a problem can be substituted. Strange as it may seem, antihistamines so widely prescribed to treat problems of allergy should not be employed topically, because they can cause sensitization in the skin and the mucous membranes. The latter possibility is cause enough to keep them out of eye and nose drops, lest they aggravate and/or exaggerate the condition they are supposed to help.

We wear clothing to protect both our modesty and our bodies from too much sunlight, cold, inclement weather, contact with irritating substances, and so on, but the very shirt on our backs can produce contact dermatitis, especially if it is made of some of the newer synthetic fabrics. Sometimes it is not the basic material of the clothing itself that causes the problem, but rather the dyes or the sizing or the substances used to create "permanent press" or other finishing materials are the sensitizers. Cotton clothing, for example, rarely causes problems, but when formaldehyde is employed to make articles "crease resistant," it can leach out with sweat to form both an allergen and an irritant. These substances tend to linger in clothing far longer than is realized. Detergents, for example, may remain in elastic waistbands, collars, and cuffs, whereas cleaning fluid can linger for some time in fabric to cause irritation. Even antistatic agents, employed to keep clothes from clumping in dryers, release chemicals which remain in fabrics to cause dermatitis. The obese tend to suffer more than those of normal weight, because they generally possess pronounced folds of fat where excessive sweating, friction, and pressure can contribute to both contact dermatitis due to the presence of allergens and to the presence of irritant factors.

Cosmetics have sent many a person to the dermatologist with an assortment of rashes, bumps, and vesicles, although considering the widespread use of beauty aids, the wonder is that there are not more complaints. The answer, I believe, lies in the care manufacturers of such products have taken to produce nonallergenic cosmetics. This is surely in their own best interests, for a customer with weeping, crusting skin does nothing for the company's image or the product's saleability.

Hair dyes have probably caused the most trouble, because they frequently contain paraphenylenediamine, a strong sensitizer. The first sign of havoc appears usually on the tips of the ears. Hair sprays, shampoos, bleaches, hair straighteners, and the like can cause contact dermatitis, often beginning on the eyelids and the ears, then appearing on the face and neck.

Lipstick can cause cheilitis, an inflammation characterized by cracking and dryness of the lips.

As the reader might expect, some kinds of eye makeup can also mar the lids as well as the general area of the eye itself. Hypersensitive women must be a little wary of their beauty aids lest they transform themselves unexpectedly to a far cry from the ideal desired. Oddly, nail polish is often responsible for contact dermatitis on the eyelids. How so? Because the nail-polish wearer scratches or rubs her eyes and because, as we have noted, the eyelids are thin skinned and prone to irritation.

Some deodorant soaps, shaving creams, and aftershaves may be responsible for contact dermatitis and/or photosensitivity. Products that contain lime appear to be the chief offenders and have a tendency of turning their hypersensitive wearers bright red and rashy when they move out into the sunlight. It is easy to imagine a clean-shaven, sweet-smelling executive smelling like a man ought to smell stepping out of his taxi on his way to a very important conference, crossing the pavement in the bright light of day, and arriving among his colleagues looking as though he had just come from a fiery weekend at the beach or, worse still, had had a three-martini breakfast. Unluckily, such a dermatitis is likely to leave a somewhat persistent pigmentation even after the initial rash has cleared. Although we physicians are generally alert to the fact that cosmetics cause allergic dermatitis among some of our women patients and are quick to attribute facial rashes and blotchy necks to such causes, we may be fooled on occasion, since she may simply be registering hypersensitivity to her husband's aftershave. Of course, the shoe could be on the other foot, and a rash-faced husband may be reacting to his wife's face powder or the like. Fortunately for cupid, these close encounters of a third kind are probably not too frequent.

This chemical and industrial age we live in is responsible for a good deal of contact dermatitis in the workplace. Metal salts, dyes, synthetic resins, solvents, alkalies, petroleum products, paints—the list is long and the symptoms produced range from mild to severe. Some of these substances are primarily irritants, and perhaps most of the dermatitis cases physicians see arise from such substances. Strong alkalies and acids are prime examples. Tracking down the cause for occupational contact dermatitis can be more difficult than one might think, because the offending agent may not be the chief material of the workplace but rather an obscure ingredient used in the manufacture of the product or even in the handling of the product itself. For a simple example, it may not be the fruit in a fruit packing house that is causing dermatitis on the hands of sorters but rather the pesticides sprayed on the fruit during the growing season. In a bakery the offending agent may not be the flour but could be the cinnamon sprinkled on the breakfast buns. Not too long ago I had a patient who was a prison guard and who suffered from dermatitis of the outer thigh. It seemed that he wore a leather holster holding a can of Mace on that side, and the can leaked a little. But since no one had ever heard of mace causing a problem, suspicion settled first on the holster, but when the patient accidently spilled a little mace on his leg, the problem was solved when a new area of dermatitis appeared.

Thus whether a substance is acting as an irritant or an allergen, the problem can be complex. The physician must lean heavily on the patient's history, with special attention to exposure and reaction time. Once suspicion appears well founded, patch testing can be employed to firmly establish the relationship. Something in the neighborhood of one in five such occupational dermatoses will be due to allergy; the rest will be the result of contact with irritant substances.

Patch-test results can vary and are not always reliable. They can be affected by a number of factors, including the size of the patch, the irritant nature of the substance (as well as of its allergenic potency that is to be tested), the skin site utilized for the patch, and even by how closely to the skin the patch adheres. There are some chemicals that are so harsh they should not be employed in patch testing. The patient must also be instructed to remove the patch (if it is a closed patch) or wash off the material (if it is an open patch) if burning or reddening of the area occurs. In spite of such faults, the patch test may be the key to whether the dermatitis is allergic in nature and what allergen is responsible while at the same time excluding irrelevant materials. The latter may be important when it comes to finding substitutes for the offending agent which the patient will be able to tolerate.

Some causes for allergic contact dermatitis are easily spotted by the physician. For instance, in the summertime I treat many a young patient whose feet have become something of an itching disaster area thanks to a combination of synthetic rubber, dyes, and sweat all come together in a pair of sneakers. I also treat a good many of their tennis-playing elders for the same reason. In much the same vein, I have a select clientele of small children who delight in building models and who react with rashes to the glue. I also treat some furniture-building elders for similar problems with glue.

Before we close the chapter on contact dermatitis, we must note that the skin often reflects the turmoil of the mind and that the dermatitis produced by emotional upset is every bit as uncomfortable and real as that caused by irritants or allergens. Some estimates suggest that about 40% of those who seek out their doctors because of skin eruptions of one kind or another are suffering from what is called psychocutaneous disease. On the other hand, skin problems in themselves have a way of being emotionally disturbing, since they so frequently alter the individual's appearance for the worse. This makes it difficult for the physician to decide which comes first, the emotional upset which may be the basic cause for skin lesions or the lesions which may produce emotional stress. Sometimes it is not easy!

Does emotional disturbance affect allergic dermatitis? Many dermatologists and allergists believe it can, and vice versa—allergic dermatitis can produce emotional disturbance. We acknowledge our realization that our skin can register emotional turmoil when we use such terms as "white as a sheet" or "red as a beet." Our skin can prickle with fear, or we may sweat with anxiety, and all because the skin is responding to stimuli from the sympathetic nervous system which, in turn, is responding to signals from that marvelous structure of the brain, the hypothalamus. The hypothalamus regulates body temperature via the sweat glands, and it responds to the part of the brain that recognizes hazard or other causes for emotional stress. Thus the skin is involved, and although emotional disturbances are not a great factor in initiating contact dermatitis and, in fact, are rarely ever a factor in producing the condition, they can be a definite factor in perpetuating or aggravating it, perhaps mainly because the dermatitis causes emotional stress and the physical conditions of that stress may in turn aggravate the dermatitis and prolong its stay. The physician must be aware of this possibility and make every attempt to alleviate such stress as part of the eventual cure of the problem.

A second factor in both prolonging and aggravating contact dermatitis is the possibility of secondary infections. It often arrives as a byproduct of the itching that accompanies most skin lesions, bringing on inordinate scratching. Children with any kind of skin problem should have their fingernails clipped short, and adults should try to maintain a mind-over-matter stance when pruritis becomes urgent. The physicians should do their best to minimize the itch of dermatitis. They will probably recommend cold water soaks, ice packs, oral and topical corticosteroids, oral antihistamines and, if infection is present, oral antibiotics. The trick is not to overtreat, for some topical medications can make matters a great deal worse, especially neomycin. Hyposensitization is not an effective therapy for contact dermatitis. Avoidance of the offending agent is the best of all preventive measures. In some individuals spontaneous tolerance does occur, especially with frequent exposure to the allergenic agent, but until it does, the only way to keep one's skin intact is to avoid. Appendix H contains some suggestions to avoid hand dermatitis.

GLOSSARY

Contact dermatitis: skin condition resulting from contact with irritants and/or allergens.

Irritant: an agent that produces (usually) local inflammation.

Pruritis: itching

Urushiol: substance in the oleoresins of Rhus plant family that is a potent sensitizer.

SUMMARY

1. Contact dermatitis can be produced by contact with either irritating or allergenic substances.

2. Symptoms of contact dermatitis range from mild rash or a few lesions to large areas of weeping and crusting skin.

3. Factors which influence allergic contact dermatitis are:

Degree of individual's hypersensitivity

Potency of the substance contacted

Duration and intensity of exposure

Presence of other allergies or emotional stress or infection or effects of sunlight or weather

4. Poison ivy is a potent and almost universal sensitizer.

5. The metals nickel, chromium, and cobalt are frequent causes of contact dermatitis, with nickel the most common of the three.

6. Drugs, especially topical preparations, can produce contact dermatitis.

7. Synthetic fibers, finishing materials in clothing, and cosmetics produce considerable dermatitis.

8. Although occupational substances produce allergic contact dermatitis, most such skin problems are due to irritants.

9. In diagnosing contact dermatitis the physician relies mainly on the patient's history, for patch testing is not always either possible or reliable.

10. Although not a primary cause for allergic contact dermatitis, emotional disturbances may aggravate and prolong skin problems, whereas dermatitis can, in its own right, produce emotional stress.

PART III

THE ALLERGY DISEASES

eleven

Asthma—with its obstruction of the airways, wheezing, a sense of smothering and fear, and, between attacks, anxiety, is an altogether unpleasant disease. Not everyone who wheezes is suffering from asthma, but some 6 to 8 million Americans do have asthma, and somewhere between 1½ and 2 million are children. The disease affects almost twice as many urban dwellers as rural and, until puberty, twice as many boys as it does girls. After this particular landmark in life the incidence of asthma evens out to remain that way until the sixth decade of life, when once again males dominate the asthma scene and have the dubious honor of outnumbering asthmatic females. The mortality from asthma and the closely related diseases of emphysema and bronchitis has been on the rise in recent years. Better record keeping, increased smoking and air pollution, and heavy industrial exposure all appear to have a role in this upward statistical leap.

From time to time asthma has been defined in various ways, for it is actually a collection of symptoms with several primary causes, although allergy is the single most common factor behind this disease. For convenience,

Asthma

asthma has been separated into two types, extrinsic and intrinsic. Extrinsic asthma, as the reader may have guessed, is provoked by influences outside the body, allergens in the main, although a number of factors can trigger and/or aggravate the disease. Extrinsic asthma can develop at any time of life, but commonly it turns up in infancy or childhood. Intrinsic asthma, about which little is understood, usually makes its appearance after the age of 35 or 40. It is believed to be influenced mainly by infection, usually long-standing infections such as those of the sinuses or other foci of infection. The prognosis of intrinsic asthma is less hopeful than it is for extrinsic, and intrinsic asthma's attacks are likely to be more severe. In truth, we do not really know what intrinsic asthma is; it is a different breed.

Asthma can be so mild as to be scarcely noticeable to patients and their families. Many people do not realize that mild wheezing can be a symptom of the disease, for they think someone must be struggling for breath to be asthmatic. On the other hand, asthma can be so severe as to be disabling, even fatal. Approximately 5,000 to 10,000 deaths annually are attributed to asthma. Childhood asthma is particularly unfortunate, because unless it is handled properly and controlled, it can warp children's emotional lives as well as their physical beings.

Asthma may be intermittent, with acute episodes followed by symptom-free intervals. Chronic asthma, on the other hand, is characterized by almost daily wheezing. The life-threatening condition of status asthmaticus is airway obstruction of a continuous nature, and it presents a difficult medical emergency to treat. It is more often seen among patients suffering from intrinsic asthma.

To understand what occurs in asthma we must know a few simple facts about the respiratory system. The nose is a familiar object, but from there on in we are in less-familiar territory. When we inhale, air travels through the nasal cavity to the larynx (an enlarged upper area of the trachea), then down the trachea, which leads into the left and right main bronchi, which, in turn, divide into smaller bronchi, which subdivide, and so on until we end with tiny airways to the alveoli (air sacs of the lungs). Capillary vessels, formed in a plexus around the alveoli, arise from branches of the pulmonary arteries. They carry deoxygenated blood from the right ventricle of the heart, and in the alveoli an exchange of gases takes place—oxygen from the air sacs for carbon dioxide in the blood. The oxygenated blood is then drained by pulmonary veins to the left atrium of the heart to be pumped to other areas of the body.

The nose and tracheobronchial tree filter out large particles of airborne

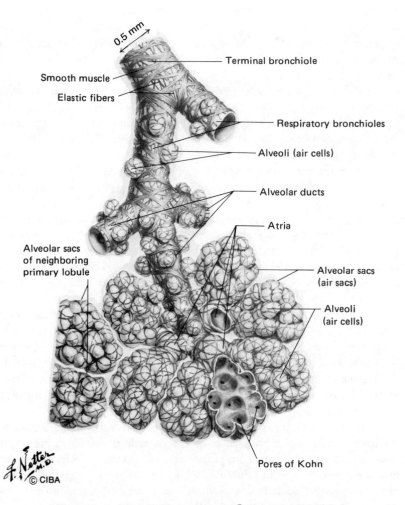

0.5 mm

Terminal bronchiole

Smooth muscle

Elastic fibers

Respiratory bronchioles

Alveoli (air cells)

Alveolar ducts

Atria

Alveolar sacs
of neighboring
primary lobule

Alveolar sacs
(air sacs)

Alveoli
(air cells)

Pores of Kohn

Structure of terminal air spaces. © Copyright 1975
CIBA Pharmaceutical Company, Division of CIBA-
GEIGY Corporation. Reprinted with permission
from *Clinical Symposia,* illustrated by Frank H.
Netter, M.D. All rights reserved.

131

debris as they warm and moisten the air inhaled. A thin layer of mucus lining the tracheobronchial tract cleanses particles that make it past the barrier of the nose; particles that do wander further and get as far as the alveoli are engulfed and destroyed by macrophages, cells that possess the capacity to surround and ingest debris and dust. Even clean air contains a multitude of particles of one sort or another. It has been estimated that a cubic foot of air can contain 3 million particles of dust, animal dander, pollen, bacteria, fungi, viruses—a witch's brew of unseen invaders which may make the reader seriously consider the purchase of a gas mask. Fortunately, the respiratory system possesses more than one means of protection. The cilia, which are hairlike projections lining the bronchi, keep up a rhythmic, wavelike motion to sweep mucus and particles upward away from the lungs. Smooth muscles that are wrapped around the bronchi can narrow the airways under the stimuli of foreign particles. At the same time, under such stimuli, the mucous glands may increase their production of mucus to wash the foreign matter from the system. In asthma, however, all this is carried beyond a normal response to invading particles. The bronchi narrow excessively, the mucous glands hypersecrete, and capillary permeability produces edema, all of which adds up to airway obstruction and a struggle not only to inhale fresh air but also to expel stale, deoxygenated air.

There is much that we don't understand about extrinsic asthma or its mechanism, but, in general, it follows a pattern of mediator release following contact of an allergen with IgE antibodies in sensitized mast cells and/or basophils, as discussed in Chapter 1. Those mediators—histamine, SRS-A, prostaglandins, and perhaps serotonin and kinins—orchestrate the abnormal responses that produce the airway obstruction. This is a simple rendition of a complex process.

Besides the factor of being hypersensitive, there are other influences, as we have noted, on the production of allergic asthma, the most important being the presence of infection, particularly of respiratory infection. Virus infections appear to be the chief villains, a conclusion which has replaced an earlier theory that bacteria provoked asthma. Frequently a respiratory infection will immediately precede an initial asthma episode, and even after the infection has been treated and cleared, chronic asthma may persist. The mechanism of virus-induced asthma is not completely understood, but it does appear that the asthmatic individual is more prone to contract respiratory infections than is the nonasthmatic person.

Asthma can also make its initial onset following surgery, especially following surgery for removal of tonsils and/or adenoids.

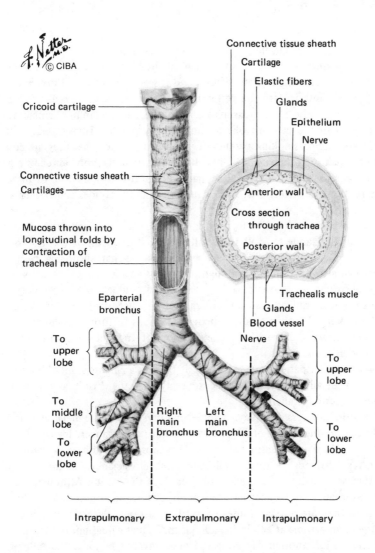

Cricoid cartilage

Connective tissue sheath
Cartilages

Mucosa thrown into
longitudinal folds by
contraction of
tracheal muscle

Connective tissue sheath
Cartilage
Elastic fibers
Glands
Epithelium
Nerve

Anterior wall

Cross section
through trachea

Posterior wall

Trachealis muscle
Glands
Blood vessel
Nerve

Eparterial
bronchus

To
upper
lobe

To
middle
lobe

To
lower
lobe

Right
main
bronchus

Left
main
bronchus

To
upper
lobe

To
lower
lobe

Intrapulmonary   Extrapulmonary   Intrapulmonary

Structure of the trachea and major bronchi. © Copyright 1975 CIBA Pharmaceutical Company, Division
of CIBA-GEIGY Corporation. Reprinted with permission from *Clinical Symposia,* illustrated by
Frank H. Netter, M.D. All rights reserved.

133

Air pollution has been a potent trigger for asthma in recent years. When massive air-pollution episodes have occurred, hospital admissions of asthma patients have risen dramatically. Dusts and gases such as sulfur dioxide and petroleum solvents irritate the respiratory system and aggravate airway obstruction. One of the cogent reasons for restricting smoking in public places is that tobacco smoke can provoke asthma. In my practice I have great difficulty in convincing smoking parents of asthmatic children that they are contributing directly to their child's ill health. Other irritants in the air can range from cooking odors to the smell of paint or varnish, from odors of insecticides to those of detergents. Even hair sprays and perfumes can trigger an asthma attack.

As noted in earlier chapters, fungi and pollens, foods and drugs, house dust and animal danders are all potent allergens and frequently are at the root of extrinsic asthma disease. Perhaps what is somewhat surprising is that weather can also be a factor, although not really a cause for the response of airway obstruction. Extremes of heat or cold, sudden weather changes, extremely low humidity, even sunlight can act as either triggers or aggravators of asthma. Very dry air may dry mucous secretions to form plugs in already obstructed airways and make the expiration of trapped air in the lungs extremely difficult.

As an aside, patients often ask me if there is a climate somewhere that is good for all allergies. I am forced to reply that there isn't, but that all climates are good for allergists!

Emotional stress also plays a somewhat mysterious role in asthma, as it does in the production of other diseases, perhaps even cancer. In fact, for a long time asthma was considered to be a psychosomatic disease brought on by "nerves." Friends, relatives, and even some physicians were inclined to agree that some asthma was "all in the head" of the victim. Although emotional disturbances influence the production, degree, and duration of asthma symptoms, they are not the causes of extrinsic asthma. Without exposure to an allergen, an asthma attack in the allergic individual would not occur. Emotional stress is just another triggering and/or aggravating factor in the "allergic load."

There is another side to the frequent presence of emotional stress with asthma. More than most other diseases, asthma breeds anxiety. The victim is truly afraid of being unable to breathe, of smothering. If asthma is severe, it is a frustrating and depressing disease. If it is mild, it is a nuisance at best. It often incurs considerable expense, and it frequently limits the patient's activities, at least periodically. Most of all, however, it frightens. It frightens the victim of an attack, and it almost equally frightens the onlooker. Thus the patient is apt to be tense and anxious, even between attacks, as are the relatives and friends, all of which makes for emotional stress.

Exercise-induced asthma has received a good deal of attention in and out of medical circles lately, perhaps because some well-known Olympic athletes have suffered from this problem. There is a paradox in this kind of asthma, for prolonged or strenuous exercise may produce an attack, whereas brief periods of activity of one to two minutes each with intervals of rest in between may even decrease airway obstruction. When groups of California elementary and junior high school students participated in the President's physical fitness program by running for six minutes, a number of exercise-induced asthma cases were discovered. Some of the youngsters had histories of other allergies, particularly of rhinitis, but some had no known allergy. We are not sure just why some people respond to exercise of four minutes or longer with bronchoconstriction. One theory is that cold, dry air triggers bronchospasm. We do know, however, that if such people inhale a drug such as cromolyn sodium or theophylline 20 minutes before exercising, the attack can be prevented.

In a somewhat related vein, although not connected with asthma, a physician has reported recently on a strange allergy syndrome induced by strenuous exercise that is severe enough to be life threatening. Symptoms are anaphylactic-like, with intense pruritis, hives, angioedema, and/or fainting (syncope). The victims in this particular report were all accomplished athletes. All required emergency treatment for this sudden and startling attack. Several did have a definite history of allergy, whereas several others had children who suffered from allergies. The majority demonstrated elevated IgE levels, but the mystery of this odd syndrome is heightened by the fact that several of the victims did not have such elevated IgE antibody levels.

If we were to compose a profile of the typical extrinsic asthmatic patient we would probably find that the first signs of allergy occurred when cow's milk was introduced into the diet. Colic, followed by eczema, would usher in the state of allergy. We would be sure to note that this baby's family had a history of allergy, at least on one parent's side and perhaps on both. As our young patient grew older, symptoms of rhinitis would develop, and in all probability he or she would suffer hay fever to some pollen or pollens or perhaps exhibit perennial rhinitis to molds or house dust or animal dander. He or she might also be hypersensitive to drugs, most likely aspirin, and might not be able to tolerate some foods. In any case, the child would be locked into step with the "allergic march," that sequence of allergy that begins with colic, moves to eczema, and ends with chronic asthma.

One physician found that 43% of his asthmatic patients developed asthma before the age of two and that 85% of them were asthmatic by the age of seven. Some allergists, myself included, believe that asthma begins fairly often during the first year of life but goes undetected by both the infant's parents and physician. In any case, when a child develops the colic-eczema-rhinitis sequence, every effort should be made to find the cause and prevent further illness, for, untreated, the "allergic march" can lead to asthma, and often does.

The initial symptoms of asthma attacks may be nasal stuffiness, sneezing, a runny nose, and a cough. Patients become restless and anxious. They generally are not comfortable lying down, but sit hunched, with shoulders elevated, arms extended as they lean forward on their hands. Their chest may hurt, the muscles of their necks standing out rigidly. They may vomit. They may grunt, sigh, or cry as they struggle to breathe air in and struggle even harder to force stale air from their lungs. Their faces usually become deathly pale. Their coughs are dry and barking, their wheezing loud and harsh. When in an obvious asthma attack, there are no or almost no breath sounds, and there is a medical emergency to face.

The thing that is so strange for family and friends is that between these seeming struggles for life itself, patients appear perfectly normal and quite healthy, their breathing free. However, they may not be as symptom free as they appear. They may be wheezing mildly, especially when exposed to cold air or when exerting or exercising. They may cough a good deal at night without, oddly enough, disturbing their sleep. Frequently, too, they display other allergy symptoms such as hay fever or perennial rhinitis, eczema, or hives.

WHAT'S TO BE DONE?

In approaching the problem of extrinsic asthma, the first step, sensibly enough, is to track down the cause. But before the hunt for allergens is on, the physician must be certain that he or she is dealing with asthma due to allergy. He or she must proceed with differential diagnosis to rule out the possibility that the patient's wheezing is due to some other pulmonary disease. In children, for instance, the first consideration might be the presence of a foreign object lodged in the throat, whereas in a much older patient, the physician may have to think about congestive heart failure. He or she must rule out the possibility of tumor or pulmonary embolism and check for a hiatal hernia. If the patient is a young adult or younger, there is the tragic possibility of cystic fibrosis. There may also be airway obstructions such as nasal polyps or enlarged tonsils or adenoids. A thorough patient's history and an equally thorough physical examination initiate this process. Chest X-rays and possibly X-rays of the sinuses may follow, along with sweat tests to rule out cystic fibrosis, tests to rule out the possibility of parasitic infestation, and nasal smears to establish whether there are increased eosinophil cells (the hallmark of allergy) and whether infection is also present.

One important laboratory test is the pulmonary function test to measure the asthmatic patient's remaining lung capacity and the degree of airway obstruction. Since a large part of the asthmatic's problems arises from the stale (deoxygenated) air that is trapped in his or her lungs by mucous plugs and constricted airways, one pulmonary function test measures the degree of the patient's expiration. The patient is told to inhale as much air as possible, which is measured by instruments, then told to forcefully expel as much air as he or she can. The results are measured on an instrument such as the spirometer, then compared with the results of the forced expiratory volume of a healthy nonasthmatic individual. The forced expiration of a given period of time, usually the first second of the test, is the measurement and is recorded in percentages. A second commonly employed test is called the "huff and puff" test, for the patient is asked to hyperventilate (breathe as rapidly as possible). The maximal breathing capacity of the total volume of air that the patient can exhale is then measured.

If possible, pulmonary function tests are made before treatment for asthma begins, both to measure the degree of airway obstruction and as a reference measurement for the effectiveness of treatment. Obviously, if the pulmonary function tests show no improvement, new methods of treatment should be tried.

Since prevention is the name of the game in asthma as it is with other allergy diseases, the physician turns to the patient's history for clues. If pollens or molds or animal danders are suspected, skin tests may help pinpoint the allergen to be avoided and immunotherapy (chyposensitization) undertaken when avoidance is not entirely possible. If foods are suspected, an elimination diet will uncover the offending agent, which can then be stricken from the menu, at least for a while until tolerance is reached to some degree. If there is a history of reaction to some drugs, the physician can prescribe a substitute.

Although preventive measures may decrease the chances of future

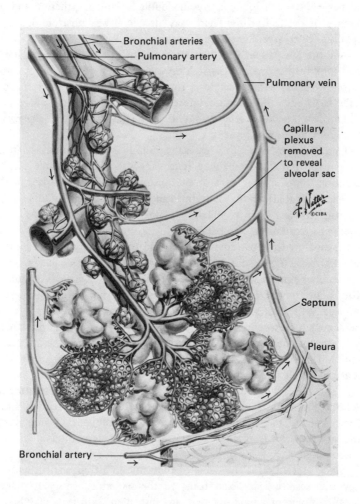

Intrapulmonary blood circulation. © Copyright 1975 CIBA Pharmaceutical Company, Division of CIBA-GEIGY Corporation. Reproduced with permission from *Clinical Symposia,* illustrated by Frank H. Netter, M.D. All rights reserved.

attacks, symptomatic treatment should be instituted for the chronic asthmatic patient. One cardinal principle for freeing the airways of mucus is adequate hydration. An adult should drink six to eight glasses of water or the equivalent in beverages each day. I tell my patients to fill a pitcher with this amount, then drain it by nightfall.

A second important step in the treatment of chronic asthma is provided by the bronchodilators, which—as their name implies—relax, dilate, and open up the airways. These are administered either orally or by aerosol (nebulizers). The latter are simple to use and give quicker relief, but they have an important drawback—they are too easy to use! This very ease of administration lends itself to overdosage, and overdosage can be dangerous. It was discovered in Great Britain, for instance, that gas-propelled aerosols of the antiasthma drug isoproterenol were responsible for a number of sudden deaths among adolescent asthmatic children.

Although oral bronchodilators are safer, they remain so, if employed on a regular basis, only when carefully monitored by the physician. A relatively new drug now in use, cromolyn sodium, is actually a prophylactic, preventing asthma attacks rather than being therapeutic during the symptom stage. It comes in a powder which the patient inhales four times a day. Its action is to block the release of mediators. It has been very effective for many patients suffering chronic asthma, helping them decrease their reliance on the powerful steroid drugs for control of their attacks.

For some patients, nevertheless, the corticosteroids are necessary, ideally on a short-term basis, for when they are employed for some duration, they must be carefully supervised by the physician. If they are precipitously stopped, status asthmaticus could result. And during times of stress, say, when the patient on these drugs must undergo surgery, dosages of the corticosteroids must be increased to handle the results of stress, because adrenal suppression is produced by long-term administration of these drugs. Alternate-day therapy with these powerful drugs has helped alleviate some of the problems inherent in the steroids, but they still create a difficult choice when employed for refractory childhood asthma, because they limit linear growth. Fortunately, newer drugs may make it possible to decrease the use of corticosteroids for such children in the future.

Decongestants and, if infection is present, antibiotics complete the medical arsenal employed to treat chronic asthma. Measures patients can take themselves are extremely important, however, in the control of this disease. No smoking, for instance, is a universal commandment for the asthmatic and avoiding the smoke of others is a necessity. Asthmatic patients should also be sure to obtain adequate rest and avoid undue fatigue. They should also avoid chilling or overheating, for extremes of temperature can trigger attacks. If strenuous exercise provokes wheezing, they can indulge in equally healthy but not quite so strenuous exercise such as swimming or walking, or they can use cromolyn sodium prior to a strenuous event to prevent asthma attacks. In general, chronic asthmatic patients, whether child or adult, should lead as normal a life as possible and be encouraged to do so by family, friends, and physician as long as the asthma is under control.

There are environmental measures to ensure such control, as outlined in Appendix B, and advice in Appendix I about how to handle weather changes and temperature problems. These preventive measures are particularly important for the severely asthmatic patient, as are the breathing exercises shown, which can assist patients in emptying their lungs of trapped air and of clearing mucus from their bronchi.

A child asthma patient should be encouraged and helped to master these exercises, for they can go a long way to restore physical well-being and alleviate potential disability.

The child or adult asthmatic patient who suffers a severe and acute asthma attack should be treated by a physician, for there is always the possibility that the patient could progress to status asthmaticus, a serious and life-threatening condition that requires immediate hospitalization and heroic measures on the part of the medical staff. This condition is sometimes defined as acute asthma that does not respond to the administration of adrenalin (usually two or three injections which appear to have no effect); in fact, the continuous attack gradually worsens.

It is well to remember that although asthma can be a severe chronic disease which can limit its victims to some extent, it need not disable them. This is wise for the parents of an asthmatic child to consider, for it is very easy to spoil a child who suffers periodic and frightening struggles to breathe. However, as nearly as possible, the asthmatic child should be treated like any other child with as few limitations as are necessary, for the child's asthma may one day be a thing of the past, but emotional development and personality are lifetime attributes. He or she should not be allowed to use asthma as a weapon against family, teachers, or friends, nor as a crutch to duck responsibility and those not necessarily pleasant but necessary chores other youngsters take on.

Once in a while a child suffers refractory asthma and no amount of a physician's care, powerful drugs, or an avoidance regimen work. It is then that the physician may recommend "parentectomy," a removal of the child

BREATHING TRAINING FOR HOME USE

Your physician has given you this booklet on breathing training so that you can help yourself breathe more efficiently. This program is designed to train your abdominal muscles to assist your diaphragm in some of the work of breathing. As you get accustomed to this different kind of breathing, you can expect to feel better and be more active in daily life.

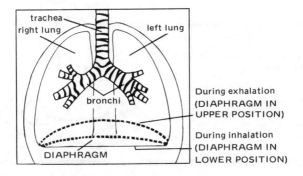

Your physician has checked the positions that are best for you at this time. The schedule of training may change as your new breathing techniques develop. Follow your physician's advice—and remember that the benefit you get from this program depends on the regularity and care with which you follow it daily.

PREPARATION

Breathing training is usually performed two to four times daily: on arising, before meals, during the late afternoon or just before retiring. The amount of time spent on each position will depend on your physician's directions.

Before beginning your training, remove tight or restrictive clothing. Be sure your nasal passages are clear. If prescribed by your physician, inhale an aerosol medication according to his directions. This will relax and open the airways in your lungs, and help to loosen tenacious mucus so it can be more easily expectorated.

Most important, do not hurry your breathing training. Rest when necessary. Hold each position as long as instructed. And in all cases, begin your day with the BASIC MORNING POSITION.

Reprinted with permission from Breon Laboratories, Inc., 90 Park Avenue, New York, NY 10016.

AT-HOME BREATHING TRAINING

Begin training sessions with aerosol
medication as prescribed by your physician

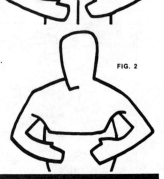

☐ BASIC MORNING POSITION

Sit erect on edge of bed or chair and
place hands over lower ribs and upper
abdomen as shown in Figure 1.
Keep shoulders down, elbows straight
out, fingers rigid. Repeat 10
times, or as physician directs.

FIG. 1

EXHALE while applying firm pressure
against ribs and abdomen with
hands. Exhale slowly through pursed lips...
lips held partly open as when you are
about to whistle.

FIG. 2

INHALE after releasing pressure of
hands slightly, but still applying effort
against chest and abdomen. Cough
gently to raise mucus.

☐ POSITION ONE

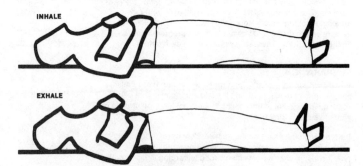

Lie flat on floor (*not* on bed) as shown, and rest left hand across chest, right hand
on abdomen. Inhale deeply through nose, letting abdomen rise. Then breathe
out through pursed lips, pressing inward and upward firmly on abdomen. Try to
move the chest as little as possible, letting the abdomen move up and down
as you inhale and exhale. As your physician directs, you may practice this way of
breathing while sitting or standing. Repeat 6-8 times. Once you have developed
this technique you should breathe in this manner even while walking.

◻ POSITION TWO

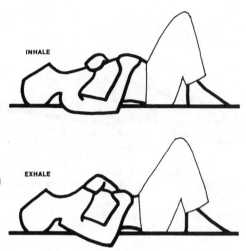

INHALE

Lie flat on floor as shown,
and rest left hand
across chest, right hand on
abdomen. Bend knees,
keeping them together.
Keep feet on floor, bringing
thighs toward chest as far
as possible. Inhale through
nose, letting abdomen rise.
Then breathe out through
pursed lips, pressing inward
and upward firmly on
abdomen. Repeat 6-8 times,
or as physician directs.

EXHALE

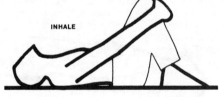

INHALE

◻ POSITION THREE

Lie flat on floor as shown, raise
knees and lock arms around legs.
Inhale through nose, letting abdomen
rise. Lift feet from floor and exhale
through pursed lips, pulling legs
toward chest as far as possible with
arms. Repeat 6-8 times, or as
physician directs.

EXHALE

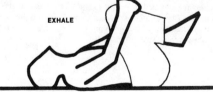

▱ POSITION FOUR

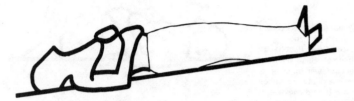

With feet elevated about 14 inches and body in a straight line as shown in illustration, rest left hand across chest, right hand on abdomen. Inhale deeply through nose, letting abdomen rise. Then breathe out through pursed lips, pressing inward and upward firmly on the abdomen. Try to move the chest as little as possible, letting the abdomen move up and down as you inhale and exhale. Repeat 6-8 times, or as physician directs.

▱ POSITION FIVE

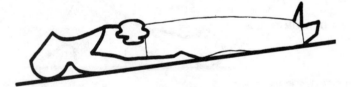

With feet elevated about 14 inches and body in a straight line as shown in illustration, place a five pound weight on the abdomen. (Use rubber hot-water bottle, or cloth sack filled with sand.) Inhale deeply through nose, letting abdomen rise. Then breathe out through pursed lips. Physician may instruct you to gradually increase weight to 15 pounds. Repeat 6-8 times, or as physician directs.

from the home environment for a period of time, usually for a year or two. Special childrens' institutions and hospitals are scattered around the country which treat just such difficult cases. Here not only is therapy constant and thorough, but whatever environmental, psychological, or emotional factors that may have been present in the home to trigger and aggravate the child's condition are absent. Personnel especially trained in the physical and mental care of the severely asthmatic child may be the most important factor in not only saving the child's life, for these children are seriously and dangerously ill, but in restoring him or her to a healthy body and equally healthy personality.

However, it is well to remember that under prompt and proper management extrinsic asthma is reversible, and permanent damage can be avoided. It is not, though, a disease to be neglected, no matter how mild.

GLOSSARY

Extrinsic asthma: asthma in response to hypersensitivity to allergens.

Intrinsic asthma: probably a result of infection of some duration, although it is not well understood.

Status asthmaticus: continuous asthma that does not respond to adrenalin.

Macrophage: a cell that ingests particles of dust and debris.

Syncope: fainting, temporary loss of consciousness because of inadequate flow of blood to brain.

Hyperventilation: rapid breathing that results in falling blood pressure, vasoconstriction, and sometimes fainting.

Parentectomy: the removal of a seriously ill child from the family environment in order to affect a cure or control of the disease condition.

SUMMARY

1. Asthma is a disease characterized by airway obstruction, although not all airway obstruction is asthma.

2. Extrinsic asthma, like other allergy diseases, is a reaction to the release of mediators when allergen and antibody IgE clash at the mast cells or basophils. The mediators, in turn, cause the smooth muscles wrapped around the bronchi to constrict, the mucous glands to hypersecrete, and blood vessels to become permeable and leak fluid, all of which narrows and obstructs the airways.

3. Factors that have a role in triggering and/or aggravating asthma are:

Infection

Emotional stress

Extremes of heat or cold

Strenuous exercise

Fatigue

Abrupt weather change

Humidity

Air pollution and irritants

4. Treatment of asthma includes drugs, avoidance measures, hyposensitization, adequate hydration, breathing exercises, and general health measures.

5. It is important that infants who exhibit the colic-eczema-rhinitis sequence be treated and controlled for allergy, lest asthma be the next step.

6. Overusage of aerosol bronchodilators can make asthma worse and even be fatal.

7. Several new drugs show promise of lessening dependency on the powerful steroid drugs to control chronic asthma.

8. It is important that asthmatic children not be allowed to use their disease as a weapon to get their own way or as a crutch to avoid responsibility. Self-reliance and independence should be as carefully nurtured for such children as for any nonasthmatic youngsters.

twelve

When I was a child I was constantly admonished "Stop rubbing your nose!" or, more sternly, "For heavens sake, use your handkerchief!" This was, of course, sometime before the universal use of tissues. As you may already guessed, I was a victim of rhinitis, more specifically, of allergic rhinitis, seasonal in nature and therefore in the vernacular, hay fever. I was exceedingly hypersensitive to ragweed pollen. By the way, in case you really wish to date me, I also had asthma, which was then treated with mustard plasters on the chest.

In any case, I was not then and am not now alone in my annual misery. Millions of Americans sniffle and sneeze in and out of pollen seasons, for as we have seen, pollinating plants are not the only allergens around. And, of course, allergy is not the only cause of upper-respiratory problems as almost everyone who has ever lived can testify. There is always the very common cold, which is so akin in appearance to allergic rhinitis that many hypersensitive souls have simply put their chronic symptoms down to "one cold after another" and damned themselves for being 90-pound weaklings. Acute or chronic sinusitis may initially look like allergic rhinitis also, but the nasal

Hay Fever
and All That!

discharge soon turns thick and yellow-green, a sure sign of infection. There is also a form of rhinitis that as far as we know has no allergy mechanism and is called vasomotor rhinitis. What we deal with in this chapter, however, is the two forms of allergic rhinitis, hay fever or seasonal rhinitis and perennial or all-year-round rhinitis.

Hay fever—which, I emphasize again, has little to do with hay and rarely sports a fever—is the most common form of allergic rhinitis, with pollens its most common instigator and ragweed pollen the most common of all. Molds, however, can shed their spores in some regions in a seasonal manner, and some insects fill the air with their allergenic debris at certain times, giving the resulting rhinitis a seasonal look. Seasonal foods such as strawberries may also produce rhinitis in the hypersensitive during their own brief span on tables. Generally, though, when we think of hay fever we think of pollen, and when we think of pollen we are apt to think of ragweed, that ubiquitous and potent weed that, as we noted in Chapter 4, springs up just about everywhere.

Perennial rhinitis may come and go throughout the year and is most frequently produced by house dust, persistent molds (especially in warm, damp climates and/or old damp houses), pollens in the Deep South (where plants pollinate all year), animal dander, foods, drugs, and some types of air pollution. Unlike hay fever, perennial rhinitis is tied to no season and may be intermittent or continuous.

Like much of allergy, there appears to be a genetic predisposition to allergic rhinitis (and to asthma), and whole families may seem to suffer from hay fever as well as other allergies. Although allergic rhinitis can turn up at any age, frequently it makes its first appearance in childhood. Many a parent has remarked despairingly to the family pediatrician, "He seems to get one cold after another no matter what I do!" In truth, it is estimated that about half of what seems to be the common cold is really allergic rhinitis, often of the perennial variety.

The symptoms are familiar. A tickling in the back of the throat that seems worse in the mornings and evenings, nasal congestion, runny nose or stuffy nose, sniffles, sneezes, constant throat clearing, postnasal drip with coughing and/or mild hoarseness, a head that feels as if it were stuffed with cotton—they all can be present and uncomfortable. Nose, eyes, and mouth may itch, sometimes intensely and especially with hay fever. The eyes may water, feel as though they had sand in them, and be red as those of an enraged bull. The ears may feel dull, full, and even painful. Some patients complain that their ears constantly pop during their bouts with rhinitis, surely a disconcerting symptom. In general, although allergic rhinitis is not a fatal condition or even a disabling one, it can be miserable and a downright nuisance. As any poor allergic soul who has ever gone for a job interview or to a somewhat formal social affair with streaming eyes, dripping nose, and a somewhat explosive and unexpected tendency to sneeze knows, rhinitis can be anything but a social asset. Snoring can also be a large problem. One wife told me that she had slept poorly for years thanks to the loud music her husband filled the nights with, but once his rhinitis was cleared, peace descended upon the home.

The human nose is a marvelous instrument. Like the mouth, it is a gateway to our interiors and as such should be pampered. It and its accompanying structures not only cleanse the air we breathe but also humidify and warm it. Tiny hairs lining the inside of the nose separate particles from the air, while mucus produced by the nose's mucous membranes raises the temperature of the air, bringing it up toward that of the temperature of the body. In the process the air is also moistened, and particles of dirt which otherwise might have found their way to the lungs are washed out. Such stuff is shunted toward the throat, where it can be swallowed harmlessly and eliminated from the body in good time. It is estimated that almost a quart of mucus flows through the nose each day, although the rate of this flow varies from one individual to another. Even so, this seems like quite a production!

The nose apparently has a cycle all its own, in which one side will become somewhat engorged and obstructed for a time, then clear while the other side takes on this temporary condition. The reasons for this taking turns at being stuffy are not clear.

Because hay fever victims register their allergies to various pollens in their season, it is important for patients and physicians alike to be aware of what pollinates when in their particular region of the country. I refer the reader back to the charts of major botanical areas in Chapter 4. Weather must also be taken into account, for a good growing season not only produces more pollen but also more severe hay fever. Thus a warm, sunny summer with plentiful rainfall produces a lush green countryside that may be a season of dread for the allergic.

In the same vein, a warm, damp spring, summer, and fall may be equally unwelcome to anyone allergic to mold.

What happens in the upper-respiratory system to cause all this discomfort, embarrassment, nuisance, and general woe of allergic rhinitis?

Unhappily for those who inherit a predisposition for allergy, the plasma cells of the mucous membranes of the nose and pharynx can produce

IgE antibodies in quantity; thus when an allergen makes its entrance, the clash can occur, releasing histamine and other mediators. The result is a response of an overproduction of mucus and dilation of blood vessels, with leakage of fluid. The former accounts for the runny-nose phase and postnasal drip, whereas the latter produces the obstruction and stuffiness. Irritated by all this activity, the nose tries to sneeze itself clear, while the throat, discomfited by all this swallowed mucus, tries to cough it up. The result is the familiar sniffling, sneezing, coughing patient whose airways are clogged, whose head probably aches because sinuses are unable to drain, and who may even be temporarily void of a sense of taste or smell and even a little hard of hearing.

Nor are the eyes immune from all this. The main symptoms of eye involvement in rhinitis are excessive tearing and conjunctivitis. In fact, in hay fever the eye symptoms may be even more severe than nasal symptoms. Such symptoms can include edema of the eyelids, intense itching, a purulent discharge (although this is somewhat rare), and reddening of the conjunctiva around the cornea. If only one eye is red and disturbed, this generally means an infection, but if both eyes are affected, allergy is usually at work.

Unfortunately, allergic rhinitis can persist for years. It was once believed that if untreated, many if not most hay fever patients could go on to add asthma to their troubles. Recent studies, however, have demonstrated that although this still can happen, it is not as prevalent as once thought. Perhaps only 5% to 10% of those who suffer hay fever move on to asthma. Still, this is enough in my view to justify the importance of treating hay fever, if for no other reason.

As with other allergy disease, a number of factors influence the severity and duration of allergic rhinitis as well as acting as triggers to produce symptoms in conjunction with exposure to an allergen. For instance, irritants such as air pollution and strong odors can trigger or aggravate allergic rhinitis. Actually, there is a priming factor, in which nasal structures, like those of the bronchial tract and of the lungs, become more vulnerable to such irritation as well as to allergens, once sensitization takes place. For example, in one study, hay fever patients were exposed to their particular brand of pollen out of its season, when their nasal structures had returned to normal. It was discovered that it took a good deal larger exposure to that brand of pollen to elicit symptoms than was required once the patient's true hay fever season had begun and his or her nasal passages were primed for allergic reaction. Apparently, IgE antibodies tend to decrease in number once exposure to an allergen ceases, and a heavier reexposure seems necessary to make them regroup, as it were.

It is also interesting to note that researchers have demonstrated that vigorous exercise can clear nasal passages and reverse the allergic response somewhat. Unfortunately, these effects are only temporary, although the person's nose may remain unobstructed for as long as an hour. However, although exercise induces constriction of the blood vessels, thus opening up nasal passages, it can also increase mucus production to warm and humidify the larger quantity of air inhaled as a result of activity. This is especially true on a cold, dry day, so the result may be the opposite of that desired. The mucous membranes may swell and obstruction occur, and, oddly enough, chilling can produce these same mechanisms, even if only a part of the body is chilled, the legs, for instance. Obviously, if you suffer from allergic rhinitis, it is difficult to win!

Even position has some influence on rhinitis. Most of us who have ever suffered thusly probably have noticed that when we lie flat, we get stuffy, but that when we sit or stand, we are apt to clear out a little.

Children who suffer from allergic rhinitis and/or asthma for any extended period of time often present a characteristic appearance that a physician can spot the moment the child walks into his office. Almost a mask, this countenance, called the allergic facies, includes dark circles under the eyes (allergic shiners), marked pallor, and a crease over the bridge of the nose which develops in about two years of using the allergic salute, an upward pushing of the nose with the heel of the hand in an effort to clear nasal obstruction. This crease differs from an inherited type seen in some families, for it disappears when the tip of the nose is pushed down, whereas the crease passed on by one's forebears remains. Often, parents of such a child never notice the crease's existence.

Diagnosis of allergic rhinitis begins with the usual thorough patient's history, for there is that initial problem of separating rhinitis due to allergy from nonallergic vasomotor rhinitis and infection, as well as distinguishing between seasonal and perennial rhinitis. Several beginning symptoms offer clues to the latter. Hay fever is generally ushered in by sneezing, followed by stuffiness and obstruction, whereas perennial rhinitis is usually heralded by obstruction and postnasal discharge. But before the physician can decide on allergy, he or she must rule out the possibility of infection and, in a small child, of a foreign object in the nose. The latter is usually characterized by only one nostril discharging matter that is very foul smelling.

Infection is the most common possibility that must be ruled out, usually by the appearance of the nasal mucous membranes and the discharge, which is confirmed by examination of a nasal smear in the laboratory. The differences between allergy and infection symptoms are indicated in the following table:

Table 12.1: COMPARISON OF SYMPTOMS OF ALLERGY AND INFECTION

Allergy	Infection (Common Cold)
Membranes are pale and boggy	Membranes are red and inflamed
Discharge is watery, thin, and colorless	Discharge is thick, yellowish
Coughing and blowing of nose is unproductive	Coughing and nose blowing produces mucus
Rarely accompanied by fever	Frequently accompanied by fever

The nasal smear will exhibit eosinophil cells in some quantity in allergic rhinitis, but few in case of infection. Sweat tests will rule out the possibility of cystic fibrosis, unless, of course, the patient is unfortunate enough to also suffer from this grim disease. A thorough physical examination will evaluate the possible role of enlarged tonsils and/or adenoids in nasal obstruction.

Abnormalities of the nasal structure must also be considered. A deviated septum and nasal polyps can cause obstruction. Nasal polyps are odd, watery, grapelike growths, which, although they occur in the presence of other diseases such as cystic fibrosis and intrinsic asthma, are probably seen most frequently among the allergic. There is also a sequence of nasal polyps with asthma, sinusitis, and aspirin idiosyncrasy. It is not known why these conditions so often go hand in hand or exactly what their relationship to each other is.

Sinus infection is possibly a cause of the polyps or vice versa. The obstruction resulting from the polyps makes proper drainage of the sinuses difficult and invites infection. Which precedes which is still a matter of speculation. And why aspirin idiosyncrasy and nasal polyps are so commonly found together is a real mystery, but it is known that once the polyps have developed avoiding aspirin isn't much help in getting rid of them. Treatment for polyps may be medical or surgical or both. Antihistamines, decongestants, antiboitics if infection is present, and possibly steroids are generally the medications employed. Hyposensitization, although it rarely influences the polyps already in ascendency, helps ensure that they will not return, for regrowth is one of their nastier attributes. If asthma is included in the prob-

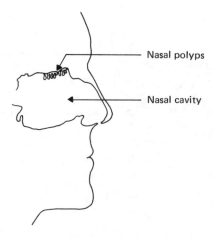

Nasal polyps

Nasal cavity

lem, antihistamines may have to be discontinued, for, as we have noted, they tend to dry secretions, worsening the problem of mucous plugs and the expiration of stale air.

Patients who do not respond to medications may have to have the polyps removed surgically. This may sound grim, but even grimmer is the fact that if left long untreated, polyps may endow their owner with a somewhat froglike appearance as the nose widens under the pressure of the growths. And that's not to mention the real possibility of sinusitis and other ills that can follow blockage of drainage and of aeration of nasal passages.

Our sinuses are something of a mystery. It is thought that since they are lined as the nasal cavity is that they, too, warm and moisten and cleanse the air. They do give resonance to our speech. The physician can get some idea of frontal sinus problems by transillumination—simply passing a light over the forehead, for instance, and if the light is diminished, the sinuses contain pus and infection.

Sinusitis is less frequently a complication of hay fever than it is of perennial rhinitis. Unfortunately, in the latter case, the two seem to run in a vicious circle with the rhinitis aggravating the sinusitis and the sinusitis prolonging the rhinitis. Through it all the victim may be feeling poorly, with an aching head or face, depending on the sinuses involved. We carry about a variety of these cavities within our heads.

One result of chronic rhinitis and/or sinusitis of some duration is serous otitis, often called glue ear. It occurs when swelling and secretions block the Eustachian tube, which normally drains and ventilates the middle ear. A

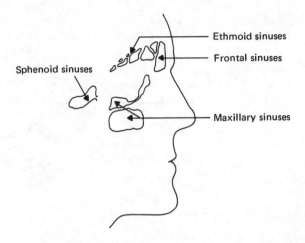

Sphenoid sinuses

Ethmoid sinuses

Frontal sinuses

Maxillary sinuses

gradual loss of hearing can occur, but often goes unnoticed. Some patients suffer disconcerting popping and cracking sounds in their ears. Happily, if treatment of the allergic rhinitis condition is begun before serous otitis has reached an irreversible stage, loss of hearing may not be permanent. It should be noted, however, that there are also other causes for this middle-ear problem.

If it remains untreated or fails to clear, allergic rhinitis can trail other unpleasant consequences in its wake. The individual may not only suffer a loss of hearing, but of taste and smell as well. A child who has become a mouth breather because of chronic nasal obstruction may take on a characteristic mouth-open appearance, which some people might designate as doltish. Whether such continual mouth breathing results in dental malocclusion and other facial abnormalities is a matter of controversy. Most serious of all possibilities, however, is that untreated rhinitis could lead to asthma.

WHAT'S TO BE DONE?

Once diagnosis has fastened on allergy as the basis for rhinitis, skin tests and/ or RAST tests plus a thorough patient's history will help uncover the offending agent. Of course, if a food is the cause, an elimination diet will be necessary to track down the culprit. If it is a drug (which is, compared to inhalant and food allergens, a rarity) the physician will have to rely in all probability on the patient's history and/or a little juggling of medications. For example, reserpine, an ingredient of some hypertensive medications, can cause nasal obstruction. Incidentally, so can the condition of pregnancy, but fortunately the problem exits as the baby makes its entrance. On the other hand, some more fortunate women find their rhinitis improves during pregnancy. The factor or factors responsible for this peculiar sequence of events remain a mystery.

Once the offending agent is found, treatment becomes a two-pronged attack: medications to treat symptoms and control measures to avoid the allergens responsible. Decongestants, antihistamines, and antibiotics, if infection is present, are employed, as with nasal polyps. When other measures fail, it may be necessary to turn to the powerful corticosteroids. Eyedrops will help relieve accompanying conjunctivitis, but many physicians will pass up the use of nosedrops, not only because they lend themselves to overusage but also because they can actually aggravate and prolong rhinitis.

The second prong of the attack, control, consists of measures similar to those employed to control asthma. Depending on the allergen involved, such measures could be the mold- and dust-control regimens outlined in Appendixes A and B, a diet which eliminates the allergenic food, removal of furry pets from the home, installation of air conditioning or the equivalent (with special attention paid to keeping filters clean), or avoidance of medications that could cause the problem. Hyposensitization for molds and pollens and even animal dander has been very effective for many patients and is well worth exploring.

GLOSSARY

Seasonal rhinitis: hay fever, symptoms seasonal in nature, depending on the presence of the allergen. Pollens are chief offenders.

Perennial rhinitis: developing any time of year, even all year round. Foods, drugs, animal danders, house dust, and molds are chief offenders.

Conjunctivitis: inflammation of conjunctiva of the eye.

Allergic facies: characteristic appearance of patient, especially a child, who has suffered perennial rhinitis or asthma of some duration.

Allergic salute: a gesture of pushing the nose upward with the heel of the hand to clear stuffiness.

Nasal polyps: watery growths in the nose which accompany some diseases and allergy.

Serous otitis: inflammation of the middle ear due to blockage of the Eustachian tube.

Eustachian tube: auditory tube that leads from the middle ear to the pharynx and drains and aerates the middle ear.

SUMMARY

1. Allergic rhinitis can be seasonal (hay fever) or perennial (all year round).

2. There apparently is a genetic predisposition to allergic rhinitis.

3. Allergic rhinitis commonly begins in childhood.

4. The nasal structures not only cleanse the air of particles of dust and debris but also warm and humidify it.

5. The eyes, sinuses, and ears can all be affected in rhinitis as well as the nasal structures.

6. Factors influencing the course of rhinitis are infection, chilling, vigorous exercise, air pollution, and strong odors.

7. Children with chronic rhinitis of long standing frequently present a characteristic facial appearance.

8. Differential diagnosis must rule out such diseases as cystic fibrosis and viral infections like the common cold before ruling allergy in.

thirteen

The human skin can register a variety of diseases, and some of the symptoms these can present on our exteriors can be horrendous. Others can be very mild, not much more than a few pimples and an itch. Frequently, to the physician's misfortune and to that of the patient, skin manifestations of disease can present a complex medical problem. Often other systemic conditions are involved, and infection is almost always a secondary consideration. Then, too, since we present ourselves to the world in our epidermal envelope, abnormal skin displays are likely to cause some potent psychological problems, especially if they are of some duration.

The epidermis is the outer layer of the skin, and its own outermost layer is composed of dead cells called the stratum corneum. The epidermis gets its blood supply from the dermis, which is laced with small capillaries. The dermis also contains the tactile cells and nerve endings which give us our sense of touch, pain, cold, and heat. Smooth muscle fibers underlie the dermis, and it is the contraction of these that makes your hair stand on end at a horror movie or a close call with a truck on the Interstate.

Skin Deep: Eczema, Urticaria, and Angioedema

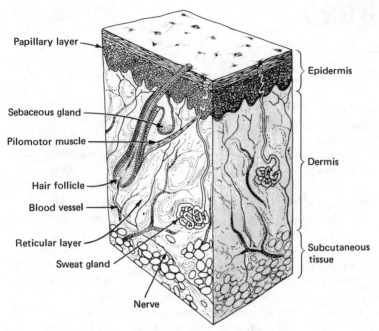

Papillary layer

Epidermis

Sebaceous gland

Pilomotor muscle

Dermis

Hair follicle

Blood vessel

Reticular layer

Subcutaneous
tissue

Sweat gland

Nerve

Cross-section view of human skin and subcutaneous tissue.

In eczema, both the epidermis and the dermis are involved. The vesiculation (formation of vesicles—blisterlike elevations of the skin, often containing fluid) appears in the epidermis, but it is apparently the vasodilation of the capillaries in the dermis which produces first the rash, then some edema as the capillaries leak fluid into the tissues. As the edema increases, vesicles form, which may rupture and ooze serum. As every victim of eczema knows full well, this process is accompanied by intense itching. If unrelieved, eczema can become a crusty, scaly mess; the skin can thicken and harden; because the pruritis is so fierce, scratching can intensify the problem by excoriating the vesicles, increasing the ooze and crust and scale and making the possibility of secondary infection highly likely. Eczema of some duration can produce lichenification of the skin, which is an exaggeration of the skin's normal folds and markings, with thickening and hardening of the skin. Oddly enough, this lichenification usually occurs when eczema is due to allergy, although there are several exceptions to this rule.

Chronic eczema will come and go, fading away to a tiny patch, only to spread out once again over large areas of the body. It does follow a somewhat standard pattern, however. For instance, in infants it generally first appears on the cheeks, then moves to the forehead and scalp and the extensor surfaces of the arms and legs. Unlike infantile eczema, later phases affect the flexuous surfaces of the arms and legs, and in adults the neck and chest are often involved, as well as the face and extremities.

It is estimated that between 1.5 and 3% of the population suffer this annoying skin problem and that about half of these unfortunates have family histories of allergy in some form. Thus genetic predisposition appears to play a large role in its development. In infants, it is most often the result of allergy to foods, with inhalants in second place. Infantile eczema may disappear by the time a child is one or two years old, or it may become worse. If it does persist, other symptoms of allergy may develop, mainly rhinitis and asthma. As we have noted earlier, this progression is called the allergic march. Eczema that makes an initial appearance after the age of two may accompany the child until puberty, when it may disappear entirely or, again, persist into adulthood. For some patients, once acquired, it becomes a lifetime proposition.

When a patient comes to the physician with wheals, welts, rashes, and vesicles, if there is a family history of allergy and/or the patient suffers from other allergies, and if the patient's own history includes some potent allergenic food or drug, inhalant, or injectant (including an insect sting or bite prior to the appearance of the problem), the physician may well suspect allergy. However, there are several other skin conditions similar in appearance to allergic (atopic) eczema. Seborrheic dermatitis is such a possibility. This is a condition of the sebaceous glands in which secretions are increased and even altered in composition, with resulting elevated patches over the skin that are bordered in red and which crust and scar. It chooses to appear most frequently over the nose, on the eyebrows, and behind the ears.

The depredations on human skin inflicted by the scabies mite may also resemble allergic eczema. As we have noted in an earlier chapter, scabies infestations come and go across the world in epidemic waves. Generally, however, scabies affects areas of the body usually not favored by allergic eczema, but when in doubt, skin scrapings will confirm the presence of the scabies mite.

Fungi and bacteria may also cause eczema, but they can usually be differentiated from allergic eczema by their appearance and, again, by the areas of the body they affect. Bacterial eczema frequently oozes a good deal, and one type forms coin-shaped plaques composed of a number of small vesicles. A yeast, Candida albicans, produces eczema generally in warm, moist areas of the body such as skin folds, and it presents a red rash with small pustule vesicles. Another fungal eczema presents a blistered appearance and usually turns up on the sides of the victim's fingers.

Allergists tend to believe that most eczema is probably due to allergy, whereas dermatologists are inclined to doubt that. I suspect that this is where the matter will rest until we know a bit more about the problem. As an example, there is one specific eczematous condition with a picturesque non-medical label of "housewife's eczema" which is generally considered to be a contact dermatitis. However, one study has demonstrated that 82% of one group of such patients either had a family history of allergy or themselves suffered from allergies. It is possible that this chronic or acute eczema on the hands of young women, for it appears to favor the young married set, has some allergy basis. The best way to control this problem is to use long-handled brushes and the like to keep the hands out of dishwater and to wear rubber gloves with cotton gloves inside (rubber can irritate) or vinyl gloves to keep the hands from contact with harsh detergents and soaps, vegetables such as onions or potato skins, or fabrics such as wool.

WHAT'S TO BE DONE?

Because inhalants play a much more important role in childhood and adult allergic eczema than in infantile eczema, the physician may use skin tests as well as an elimination diet to uncover the offending agent or agents, guided by the patient's history, for if the offending agent is a drug, such as aspirin (and especially aspirin), the clue will lie in the patient's history.

Treatment during the acute stage is largely symptomatic. Wet dressing of Burrow's solution (aluminum sulfate and calcium acetate) or even just water helps to relieve itching and inflammation. A steroid ointment may be applied, with a plastic wrap placed over the area and secured with cellophane tape. This will hasten the absorption of the steroid, but only small areas should be so treated to limit the systemic absorption of the drug. Coal-tar preparations are also quite effective in clearing up eczema lesions, but they are apt to be somewhat unsightly and quite smelly. Before applying any ointment, the cautious physician will apply a small amount of the drug to a small area to be sure the patient is not hypersensitive to the drug itself. Nor should steroid ointments be prescribed for the face, because they can create further problems.

If infection is present, and it usually is, antibiotics are employed. If possible, however, the infective agent should be cultured, for if one kind of agent is at work, a given type of antibiotic is most effective, but if another is present, a different antibiotic may be needed.

Discomfort can be lessened by wearing lightweight cotton clothing rather than those of synthetic fibers or wool, both of which are apt to be scratchy. Perfumes, harsh soaps, and detergents should be avoided as much as possible, and vigorous exercise strenuous enough to raise a sweat should be postponed until the eczema clears, because sweat can aggravate the condition. After bathing or swimming a lubricant such as lanolin should be applied to the skin over the entire body, for the skin of the eczematous patient is often very dry and the drier the skin, the worse the itch. Bath oils are also helpful and a pleasant way to relieve dryness. Care should be taken to keep the bath or shower water tepid, for if too hot or too cold it can start up itching, something to be avoided at all cost. There are soap substitutes and superfatted soaps that are helpful, although mild soaps are usually well tolerated. Lowila Cake, Aveeno Soap Substitute, Neutrogena, and Allenbury's Superfatted Basic Soap are all good possibilities. When eczema moves into the scalp or when it is accompanied by seborrhea, an antiseborrheic shampoo should be employed. The lather should remain on the hair for 5 or 10 minutes before rinsing. If the scalp lesions are inflamed, the physician probably will prescribe a steroid ointment, Topical steroid ointment does not contain sensitizing agents, as do steroid creams and lotions and thus is less apt to cause complications. Antihistamines taken orally are helpful in relieving itching, although sometimes that itching can be so severe that a mild tranquilizer may be required if the patient is to get any relief or even sleep. Loss of sleep and just plain aggravation can only add to the patient's problems in the form of emotional stress.

Which brings us to the mysterious role of emotional stress in eczema. Although we know that emotional disturbances influence skin allergies, we are not certain which comes first, the skin problem or the emotional stress. My own belief is that emotional stress is not the cause of allergic eczema but that it certainly does aggravate it, and the physical alterations such stress can produce probably do lower the patient's tolerance to allergens in the environment.

In any case, the eczematous patient should (1) follow the control measures outlined in Appendix B if an inhalant is found to be the cause of his or her misery; (2) follow a diet that eliminates an offending food; or (3) avoid the drug that the physician has pinpointed as being at the root of the problem. The wise physician and the resigned patient may well be cautious of pronouncing a "cure" when the eczema clears, for in spite of their best efforts, for some patients eczema seems to have an uncanny ability to return. Still, it can be kept within bounds.

There are several potentially serious problems that eczema can trail in its wake. One is called eczema herpeticum, which can develop when the eczematous patient is exposed to herpes simplex. The result can be mild, but it also can be severe, even fatal, with a mortality rate of 10%. A second complication is eczema vaccinatum, which can occur when an eczematous patient is vaccinated for smallpox or even exposed to someone else who has been freshly vaccinated. Fortunately, since this condition can be highly fatal for children, smallpox vacciations are now a thing of the past.

When we come to urticaria and angioedema, we find that although children commonly display these two conditions, their elders are even more prone to burst forth in wheals and welts. It has been estimated that between 10 and 20% of the population suffer from this disorder at some time. Acute urticaria, sometimes defined as hives that last six weeks or less, is most often in response to an allergic reaction, whereas chronic urticaria can be allergic or nonallergic in origin. Chronic hives, as can be imagined, can present the physician with some difficulty in diagnosis.

In this discussion, I shall include angioedema in the word *urticaria*, because their mechanisms and causes are similar. However, the reader should be aware that angioedema is marked swelling that can be generalized over a large area, even of the entire body, whereas urticaria as technically employed designates wheals, some of which can be very small and round and some of which can be quite large and irregularly shaped. Urticaria as such rises from the superficial dermis of the skin when small capillaries dilate and leak serum as a result, in the main, of histamine release. Angioedema rises in the deeper dermis from a similar process, but where vasodilation takes place in larger capillaries and fluid leakage is greater.

We are apt to think of hives in connection with our skin only, but actually they can be produced in the mucous membranes of other body systems, most commonly in the gastrointestinal tract and the respiratory system. In the former, chief symptoms are nausea, vomiting, abdominal pain, and diarrhea; in the latter, obstructed airways, especially in the area of the larynx, pharynx, and trachea. If edema is severe, such obstruction can be serious, even fatal.

As with eczema, itching can be intense, but oddly enough, on occasion itching may be the only symptom of the problem, and no lesions may appear. On the other hand, the condition can make the nicest-looking face grotesque, swelling the eyes closed and/or turning the lips inside out. The genitalia can be likewise affected.

Diagnosis depends a good deal on a thorough patient's history, skin tests and/or an elimination diet, and whatever laboratory tests seem warranted, for again, as in much of allergy, other, often more serious possibilities must be ruled out before allergy can be ruled in. Urticaria, for example, can be present in such serious diseases as leukemia or lupus erythematosus. Other somewhat common possibilities are infestation with parasites or chronic focal infection of tonsils and/or adenoids, sinuses, or even of the teeth. Young people with infectious mononucleosis may break out in wheals and itching woes, as can those suffering from viral diseases such as infectious hepatitis. Then there is a mysterious condition called urticaria pigmentosa, which begins in small children looking like ordinary urticaria, but often disappears at puberty. Equally strange but potentially far more dangerous is a condition called hereditary angioneurotic edema, which is characterized by acute and severe edema, often occurring in the larynx, where it can cause fatal obstruction. Stress, both physical and mental, extremes of heat or cold, and exertion set off this odd, nonallergic problem which differs from the physical allergy which we examine a little later in the chapter.

Once allergy has been ruled in, the hunt is on for the offending agent or agents. The physician turns detective, searching for clues among the following list of possibilities:

Foods: chocolate, eggs (especially in eczema), nuts, peanuts, shellfish and fish, milk, wheat, fresh fruit, pork, peas

Drugs: aspirin (and tartrazine), bromides, antibiotics (penicillin especially), iodides, digitalis, codeine, atropine, hormones such as ACTH, phenolphthalein (in laxatives and cake-icing coloring especially), sulfonamides, eye, ear, and nose drops, coal-tar derivatives such as antipyrine and acetanilide

Inhalants: insecticides, formaldehyde, paint, tobacco, perfume, horse dander, cottonseed, flaxseed, aerosols, cooking odors, castor beans, wheat flour

Contactants: detergents, soaps, mouthwashes, powders, hair sprays, feathers, wool, silk, clothing dyes, cosmetics, animal hair, saliva and dander, insects (caterpillars, moths, and beetles), mercury tooth fillings, mercury ointment, pollen and wax, food coloring

Insects Stings and Bites

Emotions

Sometimes it takes two or more of these factors working together to produce symptoms of allergic urticaria.

Physical allergy is a somewhat different breed of hypersensitivity symptoms. It is apparently allergic in nature and is reproducible under environmental stimuli such as cold, heat, sunlight, and pressure. Those who suffer from cold allergy, for instance, may exhibit such exotic symptoms as lips swelling so severely from sipping an icy cola or the like that they almost turn inside out, or hands all but doubling in size from handling ice cubes or snowballs. Swimming in cold water can be dangerous for such individuals, for the sudden release of histamine on contact with cold can result in hypotension (falling blood pressure). It is believed that some otherwise inexplicable drownings may be due to this strange reaction. Diagnosis of cold allergy is simple. The patient holds an ice cube to his forearm for about four minutes and the area is monitored for another ten. By this time, itching may be the initial symptom followed by a large wheal the shape of the ice cube.

Heat allergy is somewhat uncommon in children, but may turn up fairly often from adolescence on. Causes are varied:

Hot baths	Eating too fast
Exercise	Excitement
Sunlight	Overwarm rooms
Hot foods	

Urticarial symptoms of heat allergy are somewhat different from other hives, being small and accompanied by prickling, burning, and flushing. Except for those brought on by sunlight and/or exercise, most of these responses occur during the winter, perhaps because many people overheat their homes and/or pile on too many clothes. The physician may test for heat sensitivity by immersing an arm or leg in quite hot water. Oddly enough, the limb itself may simply redden, but hives will pop out over a wide area of the body.

Physicians in some cases have tried to hyposensitize patients sensitive to cold and heat by immersing a hand or foot in water of gradually increasing or decreasing temperature, depending on the sensitivity. I suppose this procedure has been successful in some cases, but it has its dangers, for an extremely sensitive patient could go into shock or suffer airway obstruction.

A few individuals develop urticaria on exposure to sunlight, especially during the spring and fall, when ultraviolet rays are greatest. This problem, however, melds into the photosensitivity that occurs in some allergic individuals who are exposed to both an offending allergen and sunlight. For a list of photosensitizing agents see Appendix J.

Another strange skin response is dermographism (*derma* meaning skin and *graph* to write—literally to write on the skin). Drawing a blunt instrument or a tongue depressor across the skin of a patient given to this manifestation will first produce a white line, then itching, then a rash and hives. The condition is thought to be allergic in nature, but its mechanism is not known. Pressure allergy is not quite the same as dermographism. It results from too tight clothing, wristwatch bands, or even from sitting too long. Although an antihistamine such as benedryl brings relief for the former, it has no effect on the latter.

WHAT'S TO BE DONE?

When symptoms of urticaria (or angioedema) are acute and severe, symptomatic treatment usually consists of injected adrenaline, which may be repeated in 20 minutes. Generally, two or three such injections are sufficient to clear the condition. If there is marked edema in the throat or severe hypotension, higher dosages may be injected or the drug given intravenously. In long-term treatment, antihistamines are helpful, especially to relieve itching. Although steroids are often helpful in short-term courses to relieve acute attacks, long-term usage should be avoided when possible.

Control measures, of course, depend on the allergen involved. If it is an inhalant, the patient should follow the measures listed in Appendixes B and C. Any offending drugs should be avoided, and if the drug happens to be aspirin, which it so often is, the patient may have to forego the list of drugs and foods in Appendix F that contain salicylates. If a food is causing the problem, the patient should avoid it for some time, then attempt to renew the acquaintance in moderation and infrequently and should consult Appendix E for plant family relationships. For some patients, hyposensitization may be effective. For others avoidance is the only real way to avoid bursting forth.

GLOSSARY

Sebaceous glands: oil-secreting glands in the skin, usually accompanied by a hair follicle.

Seborrhea: a disease of the sebaceous glands characterized by increased secretions, often altered in nature.

Lichenification: thickening and hardening of skin, with exaggeration of skin folds and markings.

Dermographism: appearance of red welts as a result of stroking or pressure.

SUMMARY

1. Eczema is characterized by a red rash and small vesicles which may ooze serum to form crusting and scaling. Intense itching is a major symptom.
2. Seborrhea, scabies, bacterial and fungal conditions must be ruled out before eczema can be attributed to allergy, although probably most eczema is due to allergy.
3. Eczema can be acute or chronic. It may appear in infancy, then disappear at the age of one or two or before puberty. Or it may arise in childhood and either clear before puberty or continue into adulthood. Often it is a lifetime problem.
4. Food allergy is a major factor in infantile eczema. Inhalant, drug, and insect allergies become factors later.
5. Urticaria and angioedema are common problems characterized by wheals, rash, edema, and intense itching.
6. Urticaria can occur in the mucous membranes as well as the skin. The gastrointestinal tract and the respiratory system may be affected in particular.
7. Urticaria can be a symptom of serious diseases as well as a common symptom of allergy.
8. Physical allergy to heat, cold, sunlight, and pressure exhibits both urticaria and angioedema.

fourteen

Gastrointestinal allergy is not synonymous with food allergy, as the reader might think. Although it is most frequently in response to food allergens, inhalants and drugs can also produce its symptoms. Those symptoms can be downright uncomfortable—abdominal pain, vomiting, diarrhea or constipation, anemia, and, in infants and small children, a failure to thrive. Some unfortunates register these symptoms in conjunction with allergic rhinitis, whereas some equally unfortunate individuals react to a food with asthma but with nary a gastrointestinal symptom. Allergy can seem unreasonable on occasion.

Often the miseries of gastrointestinal allergy are so mild and diffuse as to lead others, the family physician included, to consider the sufferer somewhat neurotic or, at best, high strung. Physicians have been known to speak of "nervous bowel," and psychiatrists to talk learnedly of patients who are unable to "digest" their emotional difficulties. On the other hand, gastrointestinal allergy can be so severe as to require hospitalization and intravenous feeding.

Colic and All That: Gastrointestinal Allergy

Gastrointestinal allergy frequently makes its first appearance in infancy and can usually be attributed to cow's milk. As one physician put it, if a 150-pound man drank as much milk in relation to weight as a baby, he would be drinking 2 gallons a day. Enough, you could say, to keep a cow busy! And as we noted earlier, cow's milk, for all its perfection, is loaded with some 20 allergens.

Gastrointestinal allergy in the infant takes the form of colic generally, with or without diarrhea. There are other causes for colic, but in our discussion here, we are talking about colic of an allergy origin. Since time for sensitization to take place is necessary, colic symptoms often wait to show up until the baby is home from the hospital and settled in, which is why pediatricians in their wisdom are wary of tinkering with the formula the baby came home with, for they are well aware that if colic should rear its constant cry, distraught parents are likely to place the blame squarely on their shoulders. And colic is a misfortune for the parents as well as the baby. It is a cruel problem, the poor infant doubles up with pain, clenches its tiny fists, turns red in the face, and screams fitfully by the hour. Fortunately for the suffering baby as well as its parents, colic generally vanishes as mysteriously as it arrived at about the age of six months. Of course, as we have noted, eczema may move in and rhinitis follow.

Sometimes a little tinkering with the formula can set matters straight. Reduction in the sugar may be all that is necessary. Or perhaps being certain that the baby is properly burped to get rid of swallowed air. Or if it's pure and simple hunger, a little additional feeding or, on the other side of the coin, if overfeeding is the problem, a little less feeding. It gets more difficult if allergy to cow's milk is the problem. Because switching to soybean formula has so often ended the nightmare of colic, many physicians in the past began to suspect cow's milk, and many now believe it the prime cause of colic. Unfortunately, so far this suspicion has defied scientific proof. Clinical experience is worth a good deal in the practice of medicine, especially when it can solve the problem even though it cannot "prove" the answer. In any case, many a colicky baby has become a happy and contented infant when soybean formula replaced cow's milk.

Alas, approximately one in five infants turns out to be allergic to soybean. Fortunately, there are other places to turn. Perhaps goat's milk will be tolerated, or a sort of synthetic milk that is predigested and contains such things as arrowroot starch, corn oil, hydrolyzed casein, sucrose, vitamins, and iron. Called Nutramigen, it may well be the answer for the infant who can tolerate neither cow's milk nor soya.

Of course, the best of all solutions is breast feeding. But before we unreservedly tout Nature's way, we must point out that the nursing mother who is injudicious about her own diet may sensitize her infant. Too many strawberries in their brief season or an inordinate fondness for cow's milk can present allergens in breast milk. Even if the mother has no allergies herself, if there is a family history of allergy on either side, she should be especially careful in her own diet while nursing, lest she sensitize her baby. I treated one small patient whose nursing mother noted that whenever she ate chocolate the baby suffered from diarrhea. This is one child who in all probability will not be able to enjoy chocolate later on.

If the mother is strict about her own diet, breast feeding is the best thing she can do for her infant for many reasons, not the least being the most important step she can take to prevent or at least delay the development of allergy in her child, especially if there is a family history of hypersensitivity. Oddly enough, allergy to cow's milk sometimes runs in families as a specific manifestation. One family studied carried this particular allergy through four generations. Generally, although allergy predisposition may run in families, hypersensitivity to a specific allergen is not so common.

Happily, in recent years the trend in America has reversed from bottle feeding back to breast feeding. If possible, the baby should remain on the breast for at least six months, for breast milk helps the infant's gut to mature, which is particularly important for the allergy-predisposed child. It is the immature gastrointestinal tract that allows allergens to penetrate to mast cells in the tract itself or to the bloodstream to contact basophils and mast cells in other body tissues, such as the skin and respiratory system. An immature gut lacks the IgA antibodies in plasma cells, which, it is thought, have the ability to counter the invasion of allergens as well as of bacteria and viruses by binding them. Breast milk provides secretory IgA until the infant's gut can produce its own.

A child who has had colic in infancy may become sensitized to food introduced later into his or her diet. Thus caution would be the watch word in starting each new food. In a later chapter we discuss a prophylactic program which, it is hoped could go a long way to prevent or mitigate the development of later allergy in such children.

When the patient exhibits gastrointestinal symptoms of abdominal pain, diarrhea, constipation, and recurrent bouts of vomiting, the physician may suspect gastrointestinal allergy, but he or she will have to do quite a bit of homework to rule out other possibilities before pointing an accusing finger. One possibility might be lactase deficiency, especially if symptoms in an infant are watery, fermentative, acid diarrhea accompanied by abdominal pain and bloating and, perhaps, by vomiting. In older children and adults, symptoms may be bloating and abdominal pain, fatty stools, and perhaps diarrhea. Lactase, an enzyme that breaks down the lactose of milk into glucose and galactose (simple sugars that are readily absorbed into the bloodstream to be metabolized by the liver), is apparently an inherited asset that is derived, it is thought, from centuries of dairying and milk drinking. Lactase deficiency is the rule among human populations rather than the exception. Of Third World peoples, for instance, 80 to 90% cannot comfortably drink milk in any quantity. Although many who have this condition, called acquired lactase deficiency, can perhaps drink a glass of milk without symptoms, more than this may bring acute unhappiness. Such people, however, can enjoy milk products that have been cultured with strains of lactobacilli, such as yogurt and natural cheeses. Acidophilus milk is now available which utilizes such culturing, or the bacilli can be added to produce hydrolyzed milk. When the bacilli reach a warm human interior, they go to work to break down lactose in the milk to a useable form.

It is interesting that most children of all ethnic backgrounds possess lactase initially, that, in fact, it reaches its peak in the full-term newborn infant, although some infants do suffer a brief period of malabsorption right after birth. By the time the child is three years old, lactase production will decline to approximately its adult level. Thus when a child inherits a low level of lactase to begin with, it will decline by this age to a lifetime production that may allow him or her to drink only a very limited quantity of milk without disturbances.

In contrast, there is a condition, which fortunately is quite rare, called congenital lactase deficiency. This problem appears as soon as cow's milk is introduced and remains as an intolerance to any amount of milk for a lifetime.

A third condition, called secondary lactase deficiency, is fairly common in infants and children. It accompanies gastrointestinal diseases such as celiac disease and cystic fibrosis, and it may appear with infectious diarrhea syndromes and in protein-calorie malnutrition. If milk is removed from the diet and the disease that has contributed to this condition has cleared, the problem is transitory. When the intestinal mucosa has recovered, milk can again be ingested with comfort.

In all three types of lactase deficiency, treatment generally consists of simply removing cow's milk from the diet, at least temporarily, and switching to substitutes such as soya. Or, as mentioned, the lactobacilli can be added to aid in the breakdown of lactose.

In addition to cystic fibrosis, the physician must consider the possibility of several other problems, such as pyloric stenosis, a narrowing of the opening between the stomach and duodenum for one reason or another; galactosemia, a disease in which abnormal amounts of galactose, a breakdown product of lactose, is found in the blood and urine; kidney disease; nervous system malfunctions; gastrointestinal malfunction; Swift's disease, an odd condition which occurs in young children with symptoms of rash, swelling of hands and feet, loss of appetite, and loss of muscle tone; or even contact dermatitis or parasitic infestation. The physician must also try to distinguish the air swallowers and the folks who apparently simply have imperfect digestion due to any number of causes which may or may not include gastrointestinal allergy. A thorough patient history often provides the necessary clues to these last possibilities. As the reader must by now realize, the causes for internal turmoil are legion.

One disease that must be considered, for a fair number of people suffer from it, is celiac disease. This condition is still something of a mystery, but we do know that wheat gluten and gliadin (a protein derived from gluten) play a vital role in its production, although its etiology remains unknown. An intolerance to gluten, it is characterized by fatty stools, loss of appetite, and a failure to thrive. It is usally seen in children ranging from six months to six years in age. Treatment commonly consists of a wheat-free, low-fat, high-protein, high-calorie diet laced with vitamin supplements.

Drugs must also be considered, for aspirin, for example, can cause intestinal bleeding and traces of blood in the stools, and some antibiotics can alter intestinal flora to produce gastrointestinal discomfort.

When all possibilities have been reviewed, the physician can think allergy.

WHAT'S TO BE DONE?

If an ingestant is suspected, the physician will turn to an elimination diet as outlined in Appendix D. Since cow's milk and chocolate (and/or the ingredients in chocolate products) have been clinically considered as most often responsible for gastrointestinal allergy, they will be the first to go. Food, of course, is not the only thing the patient may be ingesting. Chewing gum, toothpaste, mouthwash, laxatives—all such ingestants must be suspected, for some are potent allergens. Nor can inhalants be ignored; thus the physician may turn to skin tests and/or RAST to uncover such a possibility.

Severe colicky pain can be relieved with a small, subcutaneous (under the skin) injection of adrenaline when a patient presents an acute attack of gastrointestinal allergy. Tranquilizers, antihistamines, a diet of clear liquids until relief occurs, and, if necessary, IV (intravenous) fluids are all helpful in relieving acute distress.

Long-term treatment, of course, is based on eliminating the allergen or allergens responsible. In new studies, cromolyn sodium—the drug we noted earlier as being effective in preventing (not abating once an attack begins) asthma—has been found to be also effective in preventing gastrointestinal symptoms to a food allergen if taken several days prior to the consumption of the food. So far, no adverse effects have been noted to its use in this manner. Sometimes an antihistamine or Periactin, which have sedative effects, are also helpful if taken before meals.

GLOSSARY

Lactase: a lactose-splitting enzyme in the intestinal tract that converts lactose into more digestible glucose and galactose.

Lactose: a disaccharide or complex sugar.

Glucose: a monosaccharide or simple sugar that is easily absorbed and is important in the body's metabolism.

Hydrolyzed milk: milk in which lactose has been converted to lactic acid by the action of bacilli.

Pyloric stenosis: a narrowing of the opening between the stomach and duodenum.

Galactosemia: the presence of abnormal amounts of galactose in the blood and urine.

SUMMARY

1. Food allergens are the chief causes of gastrointestinal allergy, but allergy to food and gastrointestinal allergy are not actually one and the same.

2. Diarrhea, abdominal pain, vomiting, constipation, and, among young children, a failure to thrive are the most frequent symptoms of gastrointestinal allergy.

3. Colic in the infant may be the initial symptom of gastrointestinal allergy to milk, although there are other reasons for colic which must also be considered.

4. Breast feeding hastens the maturing of the infant's gut to make it less permeable to allergens, and the secretory IgA in breast milk helps the infant's gastrointestinal system fend off allergens as well as bacteria and viruses.

5. A nursing mother should be careful of her own diet, especially when there is a family history of allergy, lest she sensitize her infant by incorporating allergens into her milk.

6. An infant who has had colic may become allergic to some new foods introduced into the diet.

7. There are three general categories of lactase deficiency:

a. Acquired lactase deficiency, which is apparently ethnic in origin and suffered by most non-Northern and Western Europeans and their descendants.

b. Congenital lactase deficiency, which is a lifetime intolerance to milk.

c. Secondary lactase deficiency, which accompanies various disease states and is usually transitory.

8. Long-term treatment of gastrointestinal allergy may include an elimination diet, avoidance of food or inhalant allergens, and avoidance of certain drugs.

fifteen

When we talk about allergy of the nervous system, we are not speaking of psychosomatic or soma-psychic aspects of allergy per se but rather of actual allergic reactions that take place in the nerve tissues and the brain—the clash of antibody-allergen in sensitized mast cells and basophils. Such reactions, of course, may trail psychosomatic and soma-psychic symptoms in their wake, but the mechanism in the nervous system is as much that of allergy as eczema is in the skin or allergic rhinitis is in the respiratory system. This distinction is not always so apparent, because allergy of the nervous system so often involves feelings and behavior. Allergy of the nervous system thus often goes unrecognized or misdiagnosed.

And I must repeat, allergic reactions can occur in several body systems simultaneously. Thus the patient with eczema, say, in reaction to eggs, may also be reacting with the nervous-system symptoms of a vascular headache or even with peculiar alterations of mood. Even as it occurs in the dermis of the skin, vasodilation can occur in cranial tissue. Nor does the headache or mood alteration need eczema as a companion, for it can stand alone as a symptom of allergy to eggs or other allergens inhaled or ingested or injected.

Headaches and Behavior: Allergy of the Nervous System

Considerations of allergy of the nervous system are rather recent, in spite of the fact that Dr. I.S. Kahn introduced the theory of neurological hypersensitivity as long ago as 1927. Dr. Walter Alvarez, whose medical newspaper column of many years was followed assiduously by millions of healthy and not so healthy Americans, discussed a number of at times odd conditions arising in the nervous system which seemed somehow connected to allergy, especially allergy to foods. Allergic himself, he spoke of his "dumb Mondays," which he surmised were brought about by habitually dining on chicken on Sundays.

There is still considerable ongoing controversy about allergic reaction in the nervous system, and there is a good deal that we don't know about its possible mechanism. On top of this, its symptoms are difficult to define and to diagnose. This is especially true of such manifestations as hyperkinesis (hyperactivity) in children, as exhibited by what is known as the allergic tension-fatigue syndrome. Since many of the symptoms of neurological allergy are subjective or are reflected by the patient's behavior, scientific analysis becomes a puzzle. Yet, clinically, by employing control methods for inhalants in the environment or elimination diets for food allergens, physicians have been able to relieve symptoms of neurological allergy and to restore normal feelings and behavior. Many an allergist has been mildly startled to discover that successful treatment of a patient's allergic rhinitis also relieves the patient's insomnia, depression, or irritability. In my own practice I have had patients whose headaches are relieved when they eliminate certain foods from their menus but return when they consume those foods again.

Headache is perhaps the most common form of neurological allergy. Whether due to allergy or to other physical causes, headaches have defied precise explanation. They are commonly present as frontal pain, but they may also include the back of the head (occiput), the top of the head (vertex), and the temple area. Rarely in children, but often in adults, headaches are accompanied by one or more symptoms such as vertigo, blurred vision, nausea and/or vomiting, chills, and general malaise.

Headaches have been categorized into three general divisions: vascular, muscle contraction or tension headaches, and headaches which combine features of both.

Migraine headaches, that bane of human existence, belong in the vascular category. We are not entirely sure just what causes migraine or why, but its victims are legion. Some 8 to 12% of Americans suffer from this painful affliction, which it has been said was the thorn in the flesh of Saint Paul. Few of us have not known some poor soul who suffers from this painful condition and have not heard their tales of the agony involved. Classic migraine consists of an initial contraction stage of the arteries in the head, during which the victim often suffers disturbances—motor or sensory or mood—called the aura. Migraine patients have described auralike visions of flashing lights or zigzag strokes, much like lightning, which seem to rise behind the eyes and precede the pain of their headaches. They speak of feeling deeply depressed or of being unusually anxious or nervous. Or they complain of muscle weakness and extreme fatigue. Thus victims of classic migraine receive plenty of warning of what is to come. Old hands at the migraine game simply retire to a darkened room to wait out the storm. It could all be over within a few hours, although some unfortunates must bear their misery for several days.

The headache itself usually begins as a throbbing pain, then settles down to a dull ache. Generally it is unilateral, but about 30% of migraine victims complain of bilateral pain. Generally, too, the headache is accompanied by other symptoms of illness such as nausea, abdominal pain, a distinctly queasy feeling, loss of appetite, vomiting, or diarrhea. Patients usually become pale and feel chilled. Their behavior may also be altered, and they may become exceedingly irritable and fatigued. Visual disturbances may be present also in this later stage, such as pain on exposure to light (photophobia) and blurred and blind-spot vision (scotoma). Some victims of migraine become disoriented and confused.

Nonclassical or common migraine usually occurs without the prodromal or first-stage warnings, but somewhat diffuse symptoms such as gastrointestinal upset or general malaise may precede the headache pain itself.

Migraine typically assaults its victims from one to three times a month, arriving usually in the mornings. However, there are some lucky folks who experience migraine only a few times during their lifetimes, and others are lucky enough to suffer only mild and transitory discomfort.

Migraine headaches are thought to be an inherited predisposition, because they tend to run strongly within families. It has been estimated that the familial incidence may be as high as 60 to 90%. Frequently, it waits to make its initial appearance until after puberty, although it can occur in children. After middle age, attacks tend to grow less frequent and, for women, menopause may bring relief. However, since the reverse has been known to happen and migraine intensify in frequency and potency after this high mark in the watershed of life, this is no rule to count on.

Some allergists believe that at least some migraine is all allergic in origin and can be prevented by control measures of environmental and food allergens, especially the latter. However, research has yet to turn up a definitive link between allergy and migraine, although clinical experience seems to indicate that allergy is involved in a proportion of migraine cases.

Other factors clearly play a role in the production of this frequently fierce headache. Emotional stress appears a large factor, so much so that some physicians believe that there is a specific migraine personality—a rigid, compulsive individual who is a perfectionist determined to achieve. Other physicians, whose patients apparently do not fit this picture, dismiss any definite connection between personality and the disease, although they do not dismiss the influence of emotional stress. As we have noted, stress, whether emotional or physical, alters body chemistry, upsets the body's homeostasis (steady state), and opens the door to many ills, migraine among them. The odd thing is that migraine generally follows the climax of the stress situation and does not occur during it; thus it is a delayed bodily reaction. For instance, when I struggled through medical-school examinations, migraine turned up *after* the examinations to plague me.

Physical factors are known to play a decided role in migraine. Hormonal changes in women before the menses, during pregnancy, and at menopause, for instance, indicate a clear correlation between these states and symptoms among migraine patients. Changes in weather and barometric pressure also appear to be occasional factors, as are loss of sleep, fatigue, and fasting. Sometimes, mere changes in schedule may trigger attacks, so that the wise migraine patient learns to live by as regular a regimen as possible.

Foods and drugs both may play a vital role in the production of migraine and other vascular headaches, not necessarily always as allergens but also because of their properties as vasodilators. Foods containing tyramine, for instance, should be avoided by anyone who suffers vascular headaches, for they are potent vasodilators. Such foods are aged cheeses, Cheddar especially, pickled herring, chicken livers, cured meats such as hot dogs and salami, red wine, some beers, and alcohol in general. Monosodium glutamate, thought responsible for Chinese restaurant syndrome, should also be avoided as much as possible. And celebrating vascular-headache patients may have to do their toasting with tomato juice or the like, because champagne can go to their head in more ways than one.

Another type of headache that is somewhat different from migraine is the cluster or histamine-release headache. It is exceedingly painful and tends to arrive out-of-the-blue to last anywhere from a few minutes to several hours. Frequently it arrives at night, bringing its victim out of a sound sleep, bolt upright in bed and in intense pain. Its descriptive name, cluster, is derived from its tendency to arrive in a series of attacks, then retreat for a period before attacking in a group again.

Cluster headaches are often accompanied by nasal congestion and watering eyes. The pain commonly involves the area of the eyes, the temples, the neck, and, sometimes, the shoulders. Often the upper teeth ache as well. A thoroughly miserable condition! Men are more frequent victims than women, suffering in approximately a ratio of five to one. They are often heavy smokers in their middle years, and usually they have no family history of vascular headaches. Like migraine sufferers, they should stay away from foods containing tyramine and refrain from alcoholic beverages. One of the diagnostic tests for those strange headaches is to administer a little nitroglycerin, for it is a potent vasodilator and will almost immediately produce pain in those prone to cluster headaches.

There is also some controversy about the etiology of muscle contraction or tension headaches. Many physicians believe that they are entirely psychosomatic in origin, and they do commonly occur in response to emotional stress. They seem to accompany feelings of depression often. Whether other factors are involved is still in question. I don't believe myself that I have seen any headaches that were purely psychogenic. There always seem to be other factors involved, although trying to pin them down is rarely easy.

The tension headache is characterized by dull pain and a sense of pressure within the head. Aspirin, that universal remedy, is of little help in bringing relief. As far as is known, allergy plays little or no part in this variety of head pain.

Headaches have taken on a slightly ribald significance, perhaps because they have been employed so frequently to duck social and other events. Thus most of us approach them with an element of doubt about their reality. However, chronic headaches should be carefully checked out, for serious possibilities exist such as hypertension, tumor, or diseases such as meningitis. Less-serious complications might be simply constipation, sinusitis, or even pregnancy. Naturally, after all these avenues have been explored, it is time to think allergy. About one-third of my patients arrive in my office complaining of headaches, and the majority are relieved of this symptom by management of their allergies.

WHAT'S TO BE DONE?

After a thorough patient history is taken and an equally thorough physical examination made, with special attention paid to the various possible causes for headaches, including thyroid and blood-sugar tests and, perhaps, X-rays of the sinuses and an electroencephalogram, the physician can explore the possibility of allergy, especially to foods. The following foods appear to play a major role in the production of headaches, in addition to those containing tyramine:

Eggs	Cinnamon
Legumes (peanuts included)	Fish
Garlic	Pork
Wheat	Corn
Milk	Chocolate

Since migraine can be triggered by physical agents and gastrointestinal upsets or infection, these, too, must be considered and measures taken to relieve the last two problems. Drugs, including birth-control pills, may also be in the picture. The physician may advise the patient to keep a kind of diary of the things that are ingested, activities and moods (stress factors), physical agents such as cold and heat, and the like, with notes on whatever kind of relationship these seem to have to his or her headaches.

Medical treatment during the active phase of a migraine headache usually consists of analgesics, a sedative and/or antidepressant drug if called for, and/or antimigraine drugs. There are also a variety of preventive medications, including tranquilizers and drugs which have the property of blocking histamine and serotonin release. In general, however, long-term treatment of migraine and other vascular headaches should lean more heavily on control measures than on medications. Hyposensitization if an inhalant is the cause, elimination of the offending food or foods, and avoidance of offending drugs—all are part and parcel of prevention.

Patients can take a number of steps on their own to minimize headache attacks. Regularity in habits is one such step. Migraine patients should rise each morning at the same time and eat meals at regular intervals. They should neither fast nor overeat, for both can precipitate headache. And they should try to avoid emotional tension, a difficult task, I realize, in these somewhat strained times. One recent possibility for relieving physical and mental tension is biofeedback, a technique which trains the mind to control physical responses that are usually involuntary, such as body temperature. For example, if migraine patients can learn to raise the temperature of their hands and feet, they might be able to avert their headaches. It is thought that increasing the blood flow to the extremities can reduce the likelihood of arterial swelling in the head, which produces pain.

When we leave headaches and move to other neurological symptoms of allergy, we find a long list of possible problems, many of which are debatable, but all of which are interesting. Dr. M. Brent Campbell, who has done a great deal of work in this field, has compiled a list of symptoms he found exhibited in a group of patients. With his kind permission, we reproduce the results of his study:[1]

Headaches—allergic or nonspecific 90

Mood disturbances. 87

Vertigo 57

Gastric symptoms 46

Headaches—migraine 37

Focal or general weakness. 35

Focal or general seizures. 35

Fainting attacks (blackouts) 30

Minimal brain dysfunction syndrome 28

Myalgia (tenderness or pain in the muscles) 21

Neuritis. 13

Numbness 13

Cerebellar [symptoms] 10

Mild periods of disorganization and disorientation 9

Leg spasms. 9

Acute or chronic schizophrenia 9

Alcoholism. 9

Ocular symptoms 7

Insomnia. 6

Sleep disturbance 6

[1] "Summary of Primary and Secondary Neuro-psychiatric Symptoms of Allergic Origin in a Neuro-psychiatric Population—226 Patients." M. Brent Campbell, *Annals of Allergy*, Vol. 31, October 1973, Table III, p. 488.

It is possible to reproduce such symptoms by exposing hypersensitive individuals to their particular brand of allergens. Some allergists believe that the mechanism producing such reactions is similar to that of hives, whereas others believe that released mediators such as histamine and serotonin act more directly on nerve tissue. A good many years ago researchers discovered that when they subjected laboratory animals to anaphylactic shock, actual lesions in brain tissue developed. Other studies have demonstrated the presence of IgE antibodies in nerve tissue.

So it is not too surprising that over the years Dr. Alvarez's "dumb Mondays" have been observed in one form or another in a good many patients, especially children. Some 25 years ago Dr. Frederic Speer defined a set of characteristic symptoms of such nervous system reactions as the allergic tension-fatigue syndrome, a descriptive title for a diffuse and somewhat nebulous condition that is difficult to pin down, because it involves emotions and behavior in good part. Some allergists believe that it is entirely possible that some children who are thought to be suffering from minimal brain dysfunction are actually victims of this syndrome and that even some patients in mental hospitals or being treated for various aspects of mental illness, perhaps especially for deep depression, are, in fact, reacting allergically to something inhaled or ingested, particularly the latter. Although this, too, is a subject of heated controversy, when other aspects of allergy such as rhinitis and/or asthma are present, it is well to consider the possibility of the allergic tension-fatigue syndrome or other forms of allergy of the nervous system.

Although the allergic tension-fatigue syndrome is associated mainly with children, particularly those labeled as hyperactive, it can occur in adults, with some peculiar results. One physician wrote about a woman, who, when she ate milk chocolate, began to rearrange furniture, dust and redust the house, and, in general become obsessively compulsive, as though driven by demons. Not too long ago I treated a young girl who was normally a happy, healthy, reasonable youngster, but when she ingested raspberries, shrimp, chocolate, peanuts, or cola drinks, she became hyperactive and totally unreasonable. Her frenetic activity and mood alterations generally began within 15 minutes of ingesting any of these foods and lasted usually all day. Her own explanations of her feelings was that she felt excitement inside her and could not be still.

When adults suffer such symptoms, we are apt to put it down to some sort of personality quirk or even as a sign of potential mental illness. The notion that peculiar behavior could be due to allergy is probably the last thing friends and relatives would consider; yet it is possible. A housewife may be depressed not because she is unhappy in her marriage, but because she is allergic to the house dust she stirs up when she cleans. The business executive may be irritable and a veritable tyrant not because she is really a nasty woman, but rather because she is consuming such things as hot dogs and a cola for lunch, or, if she is really high on the corporate ladder, she may be reacting to shrimp or some other delicacy served up with her three-martini lunch. At least, if we wish to be charitable, we could consider that some adult peccadillos are perhaps due to the misfortune of being allergic.

Because the literature of allergy is replete with information about the allergic tension-fatigue syndrome as it affects children, we shall center attention on them. According to Dr. Speer, the young patient may exhibit overactive or underactive behavior or alternate between the two. Most of the attention in recent years has centered on overactive or hyperactive children, those restless little monsters who tear the home apart, drive their parents to distraction, and make teachers want to change their profession. Of course, not all hyperactivity is due to allergy; perhaps most is not, but many allergists believe that before such children are treated with potent drugs, allergy should be considered.

One of the great difficulties with a symptom like hyperactivity is finding a specific definition for a somewhat nonspecific state. Parents, teachers, and physicians are apt to have divergent views about what constitutes a hyperactive child. Many a child so labeled, if carefully watched, would seem no more than a normal child who hasn't gotten used to sitting still in a chair or at a school desk. What allergists commonly designate as symptoms of children in the hyperactive or tension phase of the allergic tension-fatigue syndrome are a frequent loss of the ability to concentrate, combined with restlessness, unusual clumsiness, irritability, and, often, aggressiveness. Such children commonly suffer sleep disturbances, cry easily, and exhibit muscle jerkiness. They may also be oversensitive to sensory stimuli—loud noises and bright lights. Like my young female patient cited earlier, they are unreasonable, uncontrollable, a disaster at home and in the classroom.

In the fatigue phase the children are listless and dull. They are usually very difficult to wake in the mornings, even though they have had more than enough sleep. They are constantly tired and may be so unresponsive in the classroom as to be considered mildly retarded. The puzzling part in all this for parents is when their children are wound up and jumping around at one time and exhausted at another. It is difficult to deal with this strange seesaw of activity and lassitude.

Are these children so different from their nonallergic peers?

In a study of some characteristics of allergic children in general versus nonallergic, one psychologist discovered that when he tested two groups of youngsters for manual dexterity, the allergic group took 129 seconds to complete the same test it took the nonallergic group only 98 seconds. In an anxiety-scale test the allergic children scored 26 versus 19 for the nonallergic, indicating that the allergic youngsters were more apt to be worry warts than their nonallergic peers. When asked to hold an ice cube in their hands until it became painful, the allergic children dropped it in 20 seconds, whereas the nonallergic group hung on for 52 seconds. Thus allergic children appear to be oversensitive and apt to be somewhat different.

In diagnosing symptoms of hyper- and hypoactivity, the physician must consider some other possible causes for such behavior. He or she must test for lead poisoning, a problem that is becoming more common in urban areas these days, and look for hypothyroidism, anemia, parasitism, malnutrition, and even mild retardation. As we have noted, symptoms of allergy of the nervous system can stand alone; thus the allergic tension-fatigue syndrome may be the only response to allergens, but it is more common to find other symptoms of allergy, especially of allergic rhinitis and asthma. Gastrointestinal disturbances and headaches also are frequent companions of the syndrome. In additon, the child may exhibit the allergic facies with marked pallor and dark circles under the eyes and may complain of muscle aches and joint pains.

As we have noted, a kindred condition exists in some allergic adults, with depression the most significant symptom. However, the depression brought on by allergic reactions in the nervous system is rarely, if ever, suicidal, as it often is in psychosis. Even so, these allergic patients frequently completely lose interest in their work, even in their families. Their appetites are poor; they suffer from insomnia; they are "tired all the time." They may find it difficult to concentrate, may be over-anxious and given to compulsive behavior. Often in adults, as in children, other allergies are present, and vascular headaches a part of the syndrome. Strangely enough, patients may suffer from a sense of unreality, and they may be extremely talkative and excitable. Abnormal attacks of yawning may overtake them, often at inappropriate times.

Studies have demonstrated a possible relationship between allergy of the nervous system and some cases of epilepsy. Dr. M. Brent Campbell has stated that neurological allergy is far more common than hitherto realized and that it should be considered as a factor in ". . . obscure and puzzling neurological and psychiatric syndromes."

WHAT'S TO BE DONE?

Treatment for allergy of the nervous system is based primarily on control measures for inhalant allergens and a diet that eliminates whatever food allergens cause problems. Antihistamines may be helpful in relieving some of the symptoms of the allergic tension-fatigue syndrome, but sedatives meant to calm the overactive generally make matters worse. It is surprising (and perhaps encouraging) how often the problem can be traced to hypersensitivity to cow's milk or chocolate or to additives, especially artificial colors, that are in some foods. In fact, the foods that are most often at the root of this problem are:

Milk	Eggs
Cola	Chocolate
Wheat	Spices and condiments

If inhalants are the offending agents, hyposensitization, if possible, and the mold and dust control measures in Appendixes A and B should be instituted.

Certainly, before we label people as "queer" or abnormal in their behavior and before we decide that the only way to control the hyperactive child is with drugs, we should make sure the problem isn't allergy, for allergy of the nervous system can be odd, and it can work in mysterious ways.

GLOSSARY

Vascular: pertaining to blood vessels.

Occiput: back of the head.

Vertex: top of the head.

Prodromal: symptoms which herald approaching illness.

Scotoma: blind gaps in vision.

Homeostasis: equilibrium of internal environment.

Hyperkinesis: excessive motor activity.

SUMMARY

1. Allergy of the nervous system is a result of the allergen-antibody clash in sensitized nerve and brain cells.
2. Allergy of the nervous system can cause symptoms of abnormal behavior.
3. Headache is a common symptom of such allergy.
4. It is thought that some migraine is allergic in origin.
5. Tyramine in some foods and alcoholic beverages is a vasodilator and should be avoided by individuals who suffer from vascular headaches.
6. The allergic tension-fatigue syndrome is most often the result of allergy to some foods and can account for at least a portion of hyperactivity in children and of depression in adults.

PART IV

SOME
CONSIDERATIONS

sixteen

The individual who is allergic to food, drugs, inhalants, and contactants may have a few special problems at home, in the workplace, anywhere and everywhere, problems that are not experienced by the nonallergic. Some of these problems can be potentially serious, for example, an asthmatic person in a confined area with a cigarette smoker. Some are on the annoying side, for example, the individual allergic to cats courting his sweetheart who happens to be a cat lover.

It used to be thought that the earliest potential problem special to the allergic would crop up in infancy when immunizations were initiated, but allergic reactions to vaccines usually crop up in later childhood, and then only very rarely. Therefore, physicians have concluded that immunizations against childhood diseases can be as safely employed for the allergic child as for the nonallergic and are equally vital for all children. As recommended by the American Academy of Pediatrics an immunization schedule would be as follows with, perhaps, minor variations (smallpox, as we have noted, has been removed from the list):

Some Special Problems

DPT (diphtheria and tetanus toxoids in conjuction with pertussis-whooping cough vaccine) and Trivalent oral polio vaccine at 2 months of age, at 4 months of age, and at 6 months of age;

Measles at 1 year of age;

German measles (rubella) and mumps from 1 year to 12 years of age;

DPT and Trivalent oral polio vaccine at 1½ years of age and again at 4 to 6 years of age;

Adult-type DT (combined diphtheria and tetanus toxoid) at 14 to 16 years of age and a booster every 10 years thereafter.

Following the above immunization schedule not only protects the child but decreases the need for potentially hazardous antisera injections in time of need, which can cause anaphylactic reactions or serum sickness, a reaction to the foreign sera in which the vaccine has been developed. Antisera are passive immunizations in which antibodies to the bacteria or viruses are developed in the sera of animals, usually the horse, and are then injected as vaccines to give immediate protection against a disease. Active immunizations with toxoids, on the other hand, are developed by the immunized individuals themselves when killed or modified bacteria or viruses are injected and antibodies created to these organisms. For example, tetanus antisera has often had to be employed after accidents in which tetanus is a potential aftermath, and many people did react to it violently, because horse sera were employed. Now, if possible, the individual is first tested for hypersensitivity to horse sera, and, in any case, the problem is mitigated because tetanus antisera is also cultured in human sera, which are far less likely to cause trouble. In most cases, if allergic and nonallergic individuals follow the recommended schedule for tetanus boosters, another booster would be all that was needed in an emergency situation. However, it should be noted that adverse reactions to tetanus boosters can occur. When they do, fewer boosters with a low-dose toxoid can avoid such problems.

It also used to be thought that measle vaccine cultured on eggs or chick embryos should not be employed for youngsters allergic to eggs, but there is some question now whether such allergic reactions even occur to these vaccines.

Occasionally adverse reactions to the pertussin antigen occur in older children, but this is a rare problem and is not allergic in nature. If use of the vaccine were to be discontinued, whooping cough would be 71 times more common than it is today. Four times as many children would die from the disease than now die from complications of the vaccination. Two deaths result from every million doses of the vaccine given.

Other reactions to DPT immunization in infancy and later are generally mild and managed by decreasing the amount of each injection and increasing the injections in what is called fractionating the dosages. Such fractionated dosages are also wise for asthmatic children and even for those who have a strong family history of allergy. The simultaneous administration of antihistamines during the immunization period will also help provide protection against hypersensitivity reactions to DPT. In any case, if a child reacts to the diphtheria vaccine, he or she probably has developed sufficient antibodies.

Oral polio vaccines and the vaccine for mumps rarely are of special concern for allergic children. Although the immunization procedure can cause problems on occasion for the allergic and nonallergic alike, these potential difficulties are generally less of an overall hazard than the diseases against which they protect. Thus every child should be immunized along the lines of the above schedule, with whatever minor alterations prove necessary.

For a number of reasons, some of them serious, surgery can pose a problem for some allergic individuals, especially when the surgery is nonelective and time is of the essence. In such cases, patient evaluation may have to be done quickly. The allergic patient could react to various drugs, anesthesia, surgical instruments (nickel), rubber in sheets and gloves, adhesive tape, and, of course, hospital food. The latter may have legions of former patients making this same claim.

The first consideration in elective surgery is whether the allergic patient is symptomatic and especially whether he or she is suffering respiratory symptoms or asthma. Even when such symptoms are absent, it is best to put off elective surgery during the pollen season for the hay-fever patient, because a flare-up of symptoms is the last thing such a patient, who is going to be recuperating, needs. It is vital that the surgeon and the anesthetist know the allergic patient's complete history and work in close cooperation with the physician or allergist. For instance, it is important that both the surgeon and the anesthetist know the drugs the patient has been taking as well as the allergens responsible for respiratory problems and whether infection or excessive mucous secretions are present.

Drug allergy is an ever-present hazard, especially to antibotics, penicillin in particular, and aspirin. They may be administered inadvertently unless care is taken to inform the medical staff as a whole of such hypersensitivity. Drug allergies and idiosyncrasies should be marked clearly on the patient's chart, preferably in red. Unfortunately, we have not, as yet, a really reliable way of detecting allergy to penicillin and must, therefore, depend on the patient's history. Before antisera is administered it should to tested in the patient in diluted strengths intradermally. Finally, since oral medications are less likely to provoke allergic reactions, they should be employed whenever possible.

When it comes to anesthesia, ether, nitrous oxide, cyclopropane, and ethylene among the general anesthesias are apparently least likely to cause a reaction, but allergic individuals, especially those who suffer from multiple allergies, have been known to react to the adjuvant drugs such as the barbiturates and muscle relaxants employed with anesthesias. Among the intravenous anesthesias, pentothal has produced severe anaphylactic reactions in some patients; unfortunately, skin tests have not been reliable in determining this potential reaction. Reactions to local anesthetics are rare and usually take the form of dermatitis. It is interesting to note that on occasion the anesthetists themselves become sensitized to some of the agents they dispense, because they frequently inhale vapors escaping in the process of anesthetizing their patients.

The asthmatic patient faces greater problems with surgery than do other allergic patients, for even if the asthma is well under control, anesthetics—whether inhaled or intravenous—muscle relaxant drugs, and the general stress of surgery may precipitate asthma attacks and pose the threat of status asthmaticus.

Another problem that could possibly face the allergic patient who must undergo surgery is if a blood transfusion becomes necessary. This is especially true for those who have a history of hay fever and/or of multiple drug allergies, for they seem more vulnerable. Symptoms of a reaction to blood transfusions might be itching, rash, hives, chills, and fever. Oddly enough, on occasion such a reaction could be to a food the donor ate prior to giving blood, a food to which the patient on the receiving end is hypersensitive.

Contrast media used primarily during X-ray diagnostic techniques may also cause reactions, especially anaphylactic shock or serum sickness. The radiopaque organic iodides, for example, have been known to produce anaphylactic shock.

The hospital setting itself must be given consideration to ensure that the patient will remain symptom free during treatment and recovery. The hospital room should be air conditioned, and nonallergenic bedding and furnishings should be supplied. There should be a no-smoking rule, both for the patient and for all visitors, nor should the patient receive flowers or potted plants. Most certainly, the patient should have no foods other than those provided by the hospital dietician, who should always be given a list of any foods the patient cannot tolerate. The asthma patient, who has more special problems than other allergic patients, should be encouraged to maintain hydration during the hospital stay. Corticosteroid drugs may have to be employed to control the asthmatic whose wheezing does not respond completely to other drugs. And those patients who are already on a maintenance steroid program for their asthma or who have received a series of short courses of the steroids (defined as six days or fewer) during the year preceding the surgical procedure may have to have the corticosteroids dosages increased. In fact, any patient who suffers from or is suspected to suffer from suppression of the hypothalamin-pituitary-adrenal axis due to steroid administration in the preceding year for any health condition should receive steroids to offset the stress of surgery. A three- or four-week course of prednisone, for example, can cause such suppression for as long as a year.

All in all, when the allergic patient's surgeon, anesthetist, and personal physician work closely together and the patient does his or her part to control the allergy, these potential problems will be minimized when facing surgery is a necessity.

The hypersensitive individual faces less potentially drastic and far more mundane problems in daily life than those of surgery and/or a hospital stay. Generally, these are problems that can be taken in stride by the nonallergic or are actually no problems for them at all. For example, travel, which is so often touted as being intellectually broadening, may be one vast headache, literally, for the allergic. Altered diet, changeable weather, and a new geographical variety of pollens and plants can pose some surprising responses on occasion. It is for this reason allergists are slow to recommend to their patients that they seek a change of residence, for there is always the possibility that new situations and allergies will crop up to new factors. The asthmatic individual, for example, may consider the sun and warmth of the desert just the ticket, only to find that the hot, dry air hardens the mucous plugs in the bronchi, making his or her condition even worse than before. By the same token, the hay-fever patient may move to an area where ragweed is all but unknown, only to become hypersensitive to some other prolific plant such as sagebrush. I think that most allergists would agree that a change of locale is less effective therapy for the allergic patient than a thorough search of the home and work environment for the offending agent or agents and careful, disciplined control measures once they are discovered. It is, for instance, all but impossible these days to escape air pollution. The stuff is generally to be found coast to coast. Nor is it easy to escape ragweed, because the more we disturb the land to make way for highways and shopping centers, developments and factories, the more we smooth the way for such weeds. In truth, home is the safest place for the allergic, even though it may take some doing to make it so.

This is not to say that vacations are out and that allergics must be stay-at-homes. It does mean that if allergics are to enjoy themselves, they will have to take some precautions, depending on the particular problems. Hay-fever sufferers should choose the time of year for a vacation least likely to provide the particular brand of allergen and areas as free of their nemesis as possible. They should carry along an ample supply of medications and watch their diets like a hawk. With food allergies, they must summon the courage to ask restaurant staffs if there is any trace of the foods they are allergic to incorporated in the meals they order. Asthmatics may have to carry their own plastic covers for bedding and perhaps their own nonallergenic pillow; they may well have to ensure that they are seated in non-smoking sections of planes, trains, and buses, then hope for compliance from the smoking public, for smokers are notoriously blind when it comes to no-smoking signs. To be charitable, perhaps they are ignorant of the hazard they pose to the health of others.

The allergic must also face up to a few sticky social problems, most of which center around parties and dining out. Let us say, for example, that you, the reader, are unfortunate enough to be severely allergic to eggs and milk. You find yourself a guest at a somewhat formal dinner, replete with rich food that is obviously the pride of your charming hostess. You are immediately faced with a dilemma, a kind of "tiger or the lady" sort of choice. Should you eat the food put before you with the sort of simulated relish it deserves, even as you break forth in incredibly itchy and blotchy hives or worse? Or should you politely explain your problem, which, in this light, may seem a reprehensible infirmity? Actually, you should have been prepared for this sort of situation, because you are an old hand at being allergic. When you received your invitation, you should have explained your problem to your hostess, offering to bring your own nonallergenic food, which could be placed on your plate in the kitchen and inconspicuously set before you at the appointed hour. Of course, your hostess could easily ensure that the menu included some things you could eat.

Yes, but what if you are the host or hostess confronted by such a guest?

Manage the above with graciousness and aplomb or, even better, serve a buffet-style dinner so that guests can pick and choose among your offerings to find the foods they can safely consume. Above all, try not to call attention to your guest's problem.

And if you are the parent of an allergic child invited to a party, again you should notify the hostess of the child's difficulties with this and that. Then, always mindful that children are in terror of seeming at all different from their peers, either provide your child's special food in a way and form that conforms as nearly as possible with what is to be served at the party or help the hostess plan some nonallergenic items your child can safely consume. It is best to remember in all this that most hosts and hostesses prefer to have their guests leave their homes in a state of adequate health.

Dining in a restaurant can be even more trying, and the more elegant the cuisine, the more hazardous for the food allergic person. It is perfectly proper, if you find yourself intimidated, to explain your problem to the maitre d' or the waiter and ask if one's forbidden food is contained in a given dish chosen from the menu. Unfortunately, there are other problems. If the restaurant is not adequately ventilated and air conditioned, cooking odors, cigarette smoke, and/or heavily perfumed ladies could do the allergic in. If dining out is an advance date and the chosen restaurant known, it might pay to call ahead to explain the problem. Probably most restaurants will happily fix you up, for they, too, have a certain dread of seeing customers leave in an obvious state of poor health.

For many allergic celebrants, holidays can turn out to be anything but happy, perhaps again from a lack of foresight. Let us start with the traditional Christmas tree. A Canadian physician, Dr. Derek Wyse, has estimated that 7% of allergic people are hypersensitive to various kinds of live trees or to the molds and whatever that accompany them into the home. Dr. Wyse found that most people reacted within 24 hours, but that some 15% of them were unaffected until the tree had been indoors for several days and had begun to dry out. He also found that mold spores in homes almost doubled with the coming of the tree and even stayed high after the tree was gone. In addition, the sticky resins of the trees had captured numerous grains of pollen blown about during earlier warm weather, and these were released in the house as the trees dried. So if you suspect that you are allergic to evergreens, and many people are, or if you have suffered in the past when the Christmas tree came through the front door, try an artificial tree and artificial decorations. It may offend your sentiments, but it will do wonders for your allergies.

As for the "groaning board" at Thanksgiving, the turkey need not be stuffed with bread—rice or potatoes or that gourmet's delight, wild rice, can be substituted. If bread stuffing is your dish, use corn or soya bread. Nor need the bird be basted with butter; suet and drippings are just as good. I have compiled a bibliography of various books and pamphlets on allergy in Appendix K, which lists substitute foods and recipes for the allergic. Some of these are especially geared to holiday meals and goodies.

Easter and Halloween can play hobs in the affairs of allergic children, for both holidays are booby-trapped with chocolate goodies, eggs, and artificial colors. Even the traditional gingerbread man of Halloween may present a problem becauses of the spices generally incorporated into its delicious form. A severely allergic small child can cause parents some anxious moments, especially if allergic to foods such as chocolate, eggs, milk, or peanut butter. Such a child loose among friends in the neighborhood at Halloween is likely to be fed these foods before attaining a necessary degree of responsibility plus the willpower to turn them down. One ingenious mother pinned a tag on her youngster to warn the well-meaning,

ALLERGIC CHILD
FOOD OR DRINK
CAN BE DANGEROUS

Older children so labeled would probably fall into a blue funk. The alernative is to teach them responsibility for their own health problems. In a way, the consequences from a failure of willpower teach a great lesson in self-control, and, since they may have to exercise such control for a number of years, parents should encourage and praise this kind of independence and self-reliance. In fact, independence and self-reliance in any child, allergic or not, should receive copious encouragement and praise.

Social problems are not the only crosses the allergic must bear, for there are certain family situations and tensions that are provoked by chronic allergy. This, of course, is not unique to allergy; it also happens with other long-term diseases. We have already discussed the fact that allergy is often so diffuse, its symptoms sometimes nebulous and hard to pin down, that non-allergic people find it difficult to believe that perfectly good food can make someone ill or that a very nice cat can noticeably shed anything into the environment to make it difficult to breathe. Allergic individuals frequently suffer the stigma of hypochondria or neurosis. They are frequently viewed with far more suspicion than charity which is tough on people who know they are not well and who feel their symptoms keenly. As we have discussed, because emotional stress can be a factor in triggering and aggravating many allergy diseases, all this skepticism can only make matters worse for allergic individuals.

On top of this, an allergic husband may find that his nonallergic wife resents having to cook special and often more difficult meals for him if he is allergic to foods, and if he is also allergic to inhalants, the effort she must make to keep house dust and mold and the like under control may fuel these feelings. Her resentment may be even worse if her favorite cat has to go. And if the shoe is on the other foot and the nonallergic husband finds himself dining on his wife's nonallergenic menu or must put up with a somewhat spartan home with few drapes or rugs or overstuffed furniture and the like or if his dog must go live in the backyard, his bitter cup may runneth over.

Allergic children can also find resentment lurking on every side, and it may be even more meaningful and harmful for them than for their elders. Siblings tend to be jealous of any special attention they may require. And when the family pet or pets must go, they will stand accused. In turn, they may consider whatever restrictions the allergy imposes as punishment, and unjust at that. They may envy siblings for their unrestricted diets and their freedom to join in the rough and tumble of the young without having to pay the piper later. Nor is it easy for parents of a severely allergic child to remain even-handed in their treatment of the family; in addition, there is some very natural resentment they may feel for the extra work special foods and special control measures require. And once such resentment surfaces, guilt follows after. There is guilt, too, when they slip up in such things as letting a forbidden item steal into the child's diet or something be brought into the home that initiates his or her symptoms. This kind of guilt can be a real burden, especially if the child has asthma and an attack is precipitated. In some families, the child's father is quick to blame the mother when the child does become ill, and this understandably makes for a good deal of parental friction plus, again, some resentment on the mother's part.

Perhaps one of the most difficult problems for parents of a severely allergic child, especially an asthmatic child, is that of discipline. It becomes a question of spare the rod and spoil or punish and risk guilt and dismay if symptoms develop. Perhaps if parents can keep in mind that the child will one day be an adult, taking into adulthood the traits and personality developed during these earlier years, they will find their way more easily through the thickets of reward and punishment. Therefore, it is my belief that parental expectations should be the same for the allergic child as they are for the nonallergic. All children should be encouraged to be independent and self-reliant and responsible. Parental emphasis should not be on the child's health problems but rather on his or her accomplishments and abilities. Probably more than most children, allergic youngsters must learn self-discipline, self-control, and responsibility for their own health problems. Raising any child is not easy, and it may be especially hard in our now ever-changing world that impinges so on the family. I think, though, that this makes it even more important to realize that what the world desperately needs is self-reliant, responsible citizens endowed with a considerable measure of self-discipline.

GLOSSARY

Toxoid: a bacterial toxin that has been treated to destroy the toxicity but retain the capacity to create antibodies. Employed in active immunization.

Antiserum (antitoxin): sera of animals (usually) who have produced antibodies to the particular organism involved. Employed in passive immunization.

SUMMARY

1. Immunization is as vital for the allergic child as it is for the nonallergic and only infrequently presents any special problems.

2. Since surgery and anesthesia may present special problems for the allergic patient, especially for those who suffer respiratory allergies, it is vital that the surgeon and anesthetist work closely with the patient's physician or allergist.

3. Drug allergies (especially to penicillin and aspirin) should be clearly marked on the patient's hospital chart.

4. Change of residence often simply exposes the allergic individual to new sensitization problems.

5. The allergic child should be encouraged to be as self-reliant, independent, and responsible as any other child.

seventeen

A large group of diseases remain mysterious in etiology and mechanism. Many of them are thought to be based on a genetic susceptibility to fail in one's recognition of self, that marvelous ability of living cells to differentiate between what is foreign and to be repulsed and what is self and to be nurtured. In some strange manner these diseases appear to be self waging war against self, as the immune system creates antibodies against its own tissue constituents. It is theorized that some triggering factor is involved—an infection or drug or some unknown environmental element. Called autoimmune diseases, they can be defined as pathological processes caused by immune responses to antigens produced by body tissues or fluids.

There are a number of theories being propounded about these diseases, many of which can be supported generally by laboratory animal models, but none has yet been clarified in human patients. As mentioned, although a genetic factor is suspected, apparently it is not the only influence at work. One theory has been suggested that these diseases might arise from a decrease in tolerance to self-antigens (allergens), perhaps because of a cross-reaction to

Self
Against
Self

tissue substances that are similar to external (foreign) antigens. Another theory has to do with a sequestered (isolated) antigen, whereas another poses the possibility that an alteration in self antigens occur to make them unlike self. A final theory suggests that alterations take place in the cells which produce the immune responses.

In any case, it is a breakdown in the immune system in which autoantibodies react with host tissue to cause considerable damage, even death. Autoantibodies are distinguished from isoantibodies; the latter are those produced by one species against antigens from another individual of the same species. An example would be the tissue rejection mechanism that has made some transplants so iffy. The autoantibody, on the other hand, is an antibody that reacts against the products formed within the individual alone. To complete the antibody rundown, we must also introduce the heteroantibody, which is produced by an individual of one species against the antigens of another species, as in serum-sickness reactions to tetanus toxoid cultured in horse sera.

Whatever the factors involved, there is apparently no single blueprint that will fit all these autoimmune diseases. We are very fond of trying to pin down the cause for something, perhaps because we feel that once the cause is known, we can avoid it like the plague or tinker with it until we fix it. Unfortunately, much in medicine is multifactorial, a word employed lately to describe the fact that frequently it appears to be the interaction of more than one causal factor which produces disease. This appears to be especially applicable to the autoimmune diseases. Two specific factors are known to have some relationship to some of these diseases—drugs and infections. One hypothesis suggests that these factors cause tissue damage, which, in turn, results in the autoantibodies which mediate the reaction. But it is quite possible that the tissue damage is a result of the autoantibodies rather than either of these factors.

Perhaps the best way to get some idea about the condition of autoimmunity is to explore several of these diseases briefly and superficially, since this is a complex subject, chock-o-block with conjecture.

Systemic lupus erythematosus (mercifully, SLE for short) is a connective tissue disease which probably presents the clearest example of tissue damage produced by multiple autoantibodies. This strange disease is more prevalent in women than in men and almost three times more prevalent in black women. It demonstrates a higher familial incidence than in the population at large, but even so, the genetic factor is uncertain. It is possible that this higher incidence within families could be the result of something similar in the environments of the victims to which members of a family are exposed.

SLE is many faceted and is expressed in multiple body systems. The most common are joint pains affecting the knees, wrists, fingers, and toes. The skin may register lesions, and a butterfly rash, the stigmata of SLE, is seen across the bridge of the nose of about half of SLE patients. Hair loss, partial or worse, may also be a feature, although it is a pleasure to state that the hair may return as therapy brings SLE under control. Since the mucous membranes may also be affected, mouth ulcers can occur. About half the SLE patients also suffer renal problems, usually mild and usually responsive to corticosteroid drugs. Some SLE patients, however, exhibit inflammation of the kidneys (lupus nephritis), which can be severe and require dialysis for the maintenance of life and/or require a kidney transplant eventually. The cardiovascular, respiratory, and nervous systems may also be involved.

Researchers have followed many a lead in their efforts to track down the etiology of this long, drawn-out, debilitating illness. One theory is that SLE is triggered by a virus, although no specific virus has been found. Another theory suggests drugs; it is known that drugs such as procainamide and hydralazine, administered for cardiac conditions and hypertension, respectively, can produce an SLE-type model. It has even been suggested that sunlight may be a trigger for some individuals, for a number of SLE patients have reported initial symptoms of the disease following a case of sunburn, and other SLE patients also suffer from photosensitivity. As in other autoimmune diseases, it is quite possible that SLE has no one specific cause but is multifactorial.

Treatment of SLE depends heavily on the steroid drugs and aspirin to contain joint pain. Antimalarial drugs are employed to control skin problems.

Early on, hemolytic anemia was considered as probably being an autoimmune disease. Characterized by an acute onset of the destruction of red blood cells, hemolytic disorders can be congenital or acquired, and it is the latter that are believed to be autoimmune in origin. Blood taken from patients suffering the congenital form of these disorders does not fare well when transfused into the bloodstream of normal individuals, indicating that the blood cells themselves are defective in this congenital form. However, blood transfused to a normal person from an individual thought to be suffering hemolysis of the autoimmune variety fares far better than it did in its owner's bloodstream, indicating that the problem is not inherent in the blood cells themselves but is rather due to something else going on in the owner's body.

Acquired hemolysis may occur as a primary disorder or may accompany other diseases such as SLE. This disease also exhibits thrombocytopenia purpura frequently. Purpura is bleeding into the skin or mucous membranes or other organs or tissues. Thrombocytopenia is characterized by the destruction of blood platelets, those small round disks floating about among the larger red blood cells which are responsible for coagulation of the blood. When they are decreased, hemorrhage can occur. Such purpura is frequently associated with viral infections, especially in children. Sometimes a decrease in platelets follows a case of measles, for instance, or even immunization for measles. It has been theorized that these disease viruses cross-react with platelet antigens or somehow alter antibody-producing cells to create a destructive antibody-antigen battle.

On occasion, the thyroid gland can be the enemy within, especially among adults. Hashimoto's disease is thought to be a result of autoantibody clash with thyroid antigen. It is characterized by inflammation of the thyroid, located at the base of the throat, and the end result can be goiter and/or hypothyroidism. The latter can lead to listlessness, low blood pressure, dry skin, obesity, slow pulse, and a general slowing down of functions. Not only is there a significant familial incidence of this disease, but it frequently accompanies other autoimmune disorders such as SLE.

A somewhat opposing problem, thyroid toxicosis, is also believed to be an autoimmune phenomenon. In this disorder, the thyroid gland appears to go berserk and overproduces its hormone, with the eventual possibility that it will burn itself out and result in hypothyroidism. The patient's pulse is rapid, and metabolism is markedly increased. Tremors, weight loss, diarrhea, and nervousness are generally present.

It is theorized that Addison's disease, in which it is thought that an insufficiency of adrenocortical hormones exists because of the destruction of the adrenal cortex, is a result of autoimmune processes, although the condition is sometimes subsequent to diseases such as tuberculosis or fungal diseases. Adrenal crisis is a serious component of this disease, but it can be dramatically reversed by the administration of adrenocortical hormones. There is also an apparent tie between Addison's disease and autoimmune thyroid disorders. This condition is called Schmidt's syndrome after the German researcher who first reported the relationship some 50 years ago.

The concept of autoimmunity has been suggested for a number of other diseases or at least as a factor in the damage they inflict. Rheumatic fever, which fortunately has been on the decline over the last 50 years in the

United States, is one such disease, with rheumatoid arthritis another. Ulcerative colitis, characterized by ulceration of the lining of the colon, is also thought to have an autoimmune mechanism, although other factors such as emotional stress, oral antibiotics, or gastrointestinal infections frequently appear to have a role.

It has been speculated that myasthenia gravis (MG), a disease with progressive muscle weakness as its predominant symptom, can be listed among autoimmune disease, because MG characteristics have been found among patients suffering other, more clearly autoimmune diseases such as SLE.

Autoimmunity offers the promise of a better understanding of such diseases as multiple sclerosis (MS) and other demyelinating diseases. These conditions of the central nervous system are characterized by degeneration of the myelin sheath (in part a fatlike substance that surrounds nerve fibers) and by lesions and hardening of the blood vessels. MS strikes mainly between the ages of 20 and 40 and, oddly enough, is more common in northern regions. For instance, the incidence in Nova Scotia is almost twice what it is in South Carolina. It is believed that a viral infection may be a factor, and there apparently is a familial relationship, but, again, this may be due to environmental influences rather than a genetic factor.

It is theorized that the increased incidence of the Guillain-Barre-Strohl syndrome that followed the swine-flu vaccination program of 1976–1977 was due, at least in part, to autoimmune reactions to the vaccine among some individuals, although the precise mechanism is not completely understood.

As the reader has probably noted from this brief and very simple discussion of a few of the strange diseases of autoimmunity, we do not know very much about them, but we are learning. These diseases are likely to be prolonged and difficult to treat. Because they involve antibodies directed against various facets of self, relief is not easily come by. Treatment is generally supportive and symptomatic. Commonly it includes drug therapy, with the powerful corticosteroid drugs as the most effective way to tackle the problem. A decrease in the immunological damage and repair of damaged tissue are important therapeutic goals. Let us hope that we are moving closer to an understanding of the etiology and mechanism of these mysterious attacks of self on self, for perhaps when we do have more definite answers, we will more thoroughly understand other still-mysterious diseases such as cancer.

GLOSSARY

Autoimmune: pathological processes produced by an immune response to antigens of body tissues or fluids.

Isoantibodies: antibodies produced by an individual of a species against antigens of another individual of the same species.

Heteroantibodies: antibodies produced by an individual of a species against antigens of an individual of another species.

Multifactorial: interaction of more than one factor to produce a result.

Hemolysis: destruction of red blood cells.

Purpura: bleeding into the skin, tissue, or organs.

Thrombocytopenia: destruction of blood platelets.

Platelets: small disks, components of the blood which release thrombokinase, a factor in coagulation.

SUMMARY

1. Autoimmune diseases are believed to be the result of antibodies developed against antigens produced by the individual's own body tissues or fluids.

2. Frequently autoimmune diseases are associated with infections, certain drugs, or some environmental factors as yet unknown, and there may be a genetic factor involved in some of these diseases.

3. Autoimmune diseases are generally of long duration, with relapses and remissions.

4. Treatment of such diseases is mainly symptomatic and supportive.

5. The drugs most important in therapy of autoimmune conditions are the powerful corticosteroids.

eighteen

Well, yes, an ounce of prevention is worth a pound of cure. I suspect that physicians and patients are in agreement with this old adage generally, but can allergy be prevented?

That's a $64-dollar question, and I am not sure that anyone can answer it with any certainty. However, there is a theory that allergy can be delayed and minimized, if not entirely prevented. Perhaps such a program is not 100% successful, but nevertheless it is well worth a try. Prevention does not come easily. It has to be worked at, but it is worthwhile, because allergy can mean chronic, sometimes debilitating illness of some duration. With families in which there is a strong history of allergy, particularly of asthma, parents should consider the regimen of prophylaxis worked out in the main by Dr. Jerome Glaser, a pioneer in the effort to prevent or at least minimize the development of allergy in allergy-prone infants. It is difficult to prove scientifically that such a program is successful; after all, it is easier to prove something that happens than it is to prove that you have prevented it from happening.

An Ounce of Prevention

In any case, here, somewhat paraphrased and shortened, are Dr. Glaser's recommendations. He begins with pregnancy, for, as he says, almost anything the mother-to-be ingests—foods or drugs—can move through the placenta to affect the fetus. Therefore, he advises pregnant women to follow these suggestions:

1. During pregnancy eat a varied and nutritious diet, but do not consume great quantities of a single food or even of a few foods. Rotate foods so that no one food dominates the diet.

2. Start a careful diet by the tenth week of pregnancy, for, as he points out, by the eleventh week IgE is forming in the fetus's blood.

3. If allergic to milk, or if there is a family history of allergy to milk, drink no cow's milk but rather use soya or other milk substitutes. Even if neither of these possibilities exist, drink no more than a pint a day of a mixture of half milk and half boiled water (boiled 10 minutes) or half evaporated milk and half water.

4. Eliminate eggs as much as possible, even if not allergic to them. Of course, if hypersensitive to eggs, then follow an egg-free diet. Dr. Glaser even advises an egg-free diet if there is a family history of egg allergy, since eggs are potent allergens.

5. Be spartan in the consumption of fish, nuts, cheese, chocolate, and peanuts, for they are potent allergens. Try not to consume much in the way of corn, wheat, and orange juice.

6. Rather naturally, eat no foods one is hypersensitive to, but also exclude those foods to which there is a family history of allergy.

7. Be guided by your physician in the matter of vitamins and calcium supplements necessary for a restricted milk consumption.

To all this, I say "Amen!" and add, "Mother, be guided by your physician to do all that you can to ensure that you will be able to breast feed your baby when he or she arrives." There is little question that this is the best of all prophylactic steps you can take, not only against allergy but against other diseases as well.

Finally, if after following all this good advice and after having denied yourself perhaps of some of the nicest of gustatory pleasures for nine long months, your child does develop allergy, do not blame yourself. This is a far from certain proposition, and there are other factors beyond a mother's control which could enter the picture after the baby is born.

And it is for this last reason that Dr. Glaser's advice does not stop at the moment of birth. In fact, perhaps the most important prophylactic measures that must be taken to prevent or delay or minimize the development of allergy in allergy-prone children must be taken during the first year of life. As we have noted, infants are more prone to sensitization during the first few months because of the immaturity of their gastrointestinal and respiratory systems and because their protective IgA antibody production is minimal at birth and only assumes a guardian role against foreign proteins somewhere around seven months of age. Thus those first few months present a clear invitation to sensitization to a variety of potent allergens. Again, breast feeding with careful attention to the mother's diet is the best of all protections, for, clearly, breast milk was designed by nature for the immature human gut. It should be continued for at least four months, preferably for six.

Sometimes, however, for one reason or another, formula must be employed. The allergy-prone infant should not be given cow's milk, and even when it does enter the child's life later on, it should do so initially in a heat-treated form. Soya formula is preferable for the baby whose family has a history of allergy, but since one in five infants is also allergic to soybean, a meat-based or other substitute formula as suggested by the pediatrician may have to be employed.

Baby food manufacturers have gotten out their products in cute little jars that are just about irresistible to mothers eager to ensure that baby's stomach is full and that they both will be able to sleep the night through. American babies during the last few decades have been started on solid foods earlier and earlier. This is unfortunate for the allergy-prone baby, who should not have solid foods until at least three months of age, and then should be given cereals such as rice, oats, or barley. Rice is the least likely to cause any problems, and wheat and corn should wait a bit, because they are potent allergens.

At five to six months fruits and vegetables can be added, but always one at a time, with an interval of three days between the introduction of each new food. Pears and apricots are the least allergenic fruits, with mushed up bananas a good third, if the first two go down without incident. Citrus fruits should wait until the allergy-prone baby is at least a year old, and berries should arrive in the menu only after the second birthday rolls around. The child's pediatrician will probably recommend ascorbic acid to provide the necessary vitamin C.

Carrots, beets, squash, and sweet potatoes are the least allergenic vegetables. Legumes, such as peas and beans (and peanuts, lest the reader forget that they, too, are a legume), should wait until the baby is a year old, for they can be potent allergens. In spite of Popeye, spinach, too, should wait until the baby is a yearling, for it can irritate the skin, especially around the mouth, as well as sensitize.

Eggs should not be introduced into the diet until the baby is at least nine months old, preferably a year old, and then only in small amounts of hardboiled yolk which are gradually increased until the baby is consuming the whole yolk without problems. When three yolks a week go down and the baby is still well and happy, a little of the hardboiled white can be added. It, too, should be increased gradually in amount until the whole egg is being consumed. When three eggs a week in all their hardboiled glory are being eaten without untoward incidents, it can be concluded that baby has not been sensitized to this strongly allergenic but highly nutritious food. Eggs can then be served in any fashion, but, please, with moderation. Everything should be in moderation for the allergy prone.

All things considered, for the nonallergic baby as well as for the allergy prone, there is little to be gained by rushing to a solid diet.

When the baby is eight or nine months old, soybean milk can be cautiously put aside and evaporated milk tried. If all goes well, pasteurized cow's milk may then be tolerated.

Diet, of course, is not the only aspect of an allergy-prevention program. Environmental-control measures must also be considered, because inhalant allergens can sensitize, especially as the child grows older. All things of feather and fur, animate or inanimate, should not dwell under the same roof as an allergy-prone child. Mold- and house-dust control measures as outlined in Appendixes A and B should be instituted.

Since many of these control measures mean considerable added work for parents, especially mothers and especially in families with other children, can we assess their effectiveness?

Dr. Glaser conducted a study himself of newborn infants who were allergy prone. He followed one group of 96 infants whose mothers had followed a restricted diet low in milk and eggs both during pregnancy and the nursing period. The babies received no cow's milk, and their supplemental formula was either soybean or meat-based milk. A second group was made up of the siblings, but this time the mothers had not been on a controlled diet during their fetal and infant periods. This sibling group had received cow's milk from infancy. A control group of children was unrelated to the first two and had also received cow's milk and were also allergy prone. The results of this study as reported by Dr. Glaser indicated that the children on his controlled, prophylactic program developed approximately 25% fewer allergies than their siblings or youngsters in the unrelated third group.

Dr. Glaser goes on to buttress the value of his regimen with a discussion about a group of Tokelau Islanders who were evacuated to New Zealand after their homes were destroyed by a hurricane. Ordinarily, Islander mothers breast fed their infants as a matter of course for as long as a year with only very late additions of other foods. Allergy among these children was rare in their native home. But after they had resided in New Zealand for some time and had begun to follow the customs of their new home by adding cow's milk to their infants' diets, allergies became frequent among the children.

It must be said, however, that other studies were not so conclusive as to the value of this regimen. Other groups of children studied have turned up with approximately the same incidence of allergy as youngsters on unrestricted, uncontrolled diets, with, it is important to note, the exception of those children who were breast fed in infancy. These children nursed Nature's way appear to develop allergy at a later age, if they develop it at all.

My own judgment in this, and it is based wholly on my clinical experience as an allergist, is that (1) breast feeding confers a tremendous advantage for the infant's health in general and may well defer and/or minimize any later development of allergy, if not prevent it; (2) Dr. Glaser's program is nutritious and may very well help the allergy-prone child; and (3) when there is a family history of allergy, this diet is well worth the effort. I would add here that great care should be taken not to include allergenic foods in the diet or expose the child to inhalant allergens when the child is ill or even during the convalescent period, for, as we have noted, infection often opens the door to allergy. Many a viral infection during the first year of life has been a precursor of allergy. During and immediately following an illness or even immunization against an illness is a period of special vulnerability.

Finally, I wish to emphasize that if the reader contemplates following Dr. Glaser's regimen or any of my various bits of wisdom tossed out in this book, he or she should consult his or her own physician before applying this assorted wisdom, for there may be other considerations and other health problems which must be taken into account. Nothing written here is intended as a do-it-yourself program. Rather, it is meant to enlighten. And I hope it has.

APPENDIXES

APPENDIX A:
MOLD CONTROL MEASURES

Places Where Molds Are Found

1. Gardens
2. Farms
3. Certain occupations (A) carpenters, (B) bakers, (C) florists, (D) farmers, (E) paper hangers, (F) mill workers, (G) mattress upholstery work.
4. Summer cottages
5. Grain bins
6. On potted plants and leaves
7. Some foods: (A) cheese, (B) bread, (C) yeast, (D) decayed foods
8. Damp closets
9. Mattresses
10. On some grasses and weeds
11. Shoes and clothing in closets

Molds grow best in warm, moist places and grow on nearly anything except metals. They grow on feathers, trees, plants, cellulose, and they may be outside or inside the house. They occur all year round, but some molds have a seasonal incidence. Some molds are found more just after frost occurs and when the leaves fall.

To Avoid Molds

1. Avoid damp basements.
2. Avoid being out in a storm.
3. Avoid occupations where molds are found such as: paper hanging, mill working, mattress upholstering, antique and furniture dealers, etc.
4. Avoid foods with molds on them such as cheese, moldy bread, yeast, and decayed foods.

5. Follow dust and feather control measures.

6. Keep luggage dry and waxed.

7. Change furnace filters.

8. Check drainage systems.

9. Avoid cleaning out leaves in the fall and cutting grass in the summer.

10. If you use a summer cottage have it aired out well before going inside.

APPENDIX B:
PREPARATION AND MAINTENANCE
OF A DUST-FREE HOUSE

House dust is the fine dust which is formed by the aging of materials which make up household articles, furniture, and clothing. It is the fine lint and dust from mattresses, pillows, upholstered furniture, drapes, curtains, rugs, bedspreads, blankets, quilts, closets, chests, drawers, books, papers, sweaters, and other clothing. Furniture and furnishings are likely to have much lint. Dust develops in stored articles and in furniture as they become older. During the aging process the substance composing these articles deteriorates into a fine dust.

Street dust is entirely different from house dust. Your cooperation in controlling the amount of house dust you inhale will be of tremendous benefit to you. We cannot urge you too strongly the importance of carrying out the house-dust avoidance instructions which follow.

Bedroom

1. The room must be completely emptied, just as if you were moving. Give the room a thorough cleaning and scrubbing to eliminate all traces of dust. Clean walls, wash down if possible. Scrub the woodwork, floors, baseboards, closets, etc. Every inch of exposed or hidden surface must be spic and span. Floors or linoleum should then be oiled or waxed. Linoleum,

if used, should be cemented to the floor. Rag rugs may be used on the floor. These should be washed weekly.

2. Cleaning should be done only when the patient is out of the room.

3. Outside the room, clean every inch of the bed. Scrub the bed and open coil springs. Bed and coil springs should be cleaned every two weeks. If the same mattress and box springs are to be used, each should be encased with an allergic dust-proof cover. Merely clean with a damp, soapy cloth and wipe dry. If you have a sleep sentry dust-proof mattress and box springs no special covers are required. Ordinary pillows must be made dust proof with special coverings and zippers sealed with adhesive tape for maximum protection. A dust-free pillow with special coverings may be used in the room. Rubber foam pillows may be used. If two beds are to be used in the room, both must be prepared identically.

4. Use only freshly laundered linens, washable cotton spreads, woolen blankets (not the fuzzy kind.) If you are sensitive to wool, use ordinary cotton blankets. Blankets and spreads should be washed at least once a month. Avoid blankets that have not been washed. Plain light curtains or Venetian blinds may be used on the windows. Wash them weekly. Scrubbed wooden or metal chairs, or chairs covered with leather or leatherette may be used in this room. Upholstered furniture is taboo.

5. Clothing must be stored outside the room. Dressing and undressing should be done in another room.

Keep all pets out of the room and the house, especially dogs and cats. Canaries, parrots, and pigeons are not allowed as pets.

Screens, ventilators, or anything that helps keep out dust and pollens are desirable. Use only insecticides and cosmetics approved by your doctor.

6. The temperature of this room, when occupied, should always be above 65 degrees, particularly at night. Determine the temperature of this room by means of a wall thermometer.

Steam or hot water heat is preferable to hot air heat. An electric heater or a good gas heater may be used. If furnace heat outlets exist, a dust filter must be installed and the filter changed frequently. When not in use, furnance pipe outlets should be sealed with a dust-proof fabric held intact with adhesive. Holes or cracks in the floor or walls should be sealed.

7. This room should be cleaned daily and thoroughly cleaned weekly. Do it while the patient is out of the room. If the patient must clean his or her own room a gauze mask should be worn. After cleaning, shut the windows and doors for an hour or two before the patient is ready to occupy the room.

Guide to "desensitizing" a room

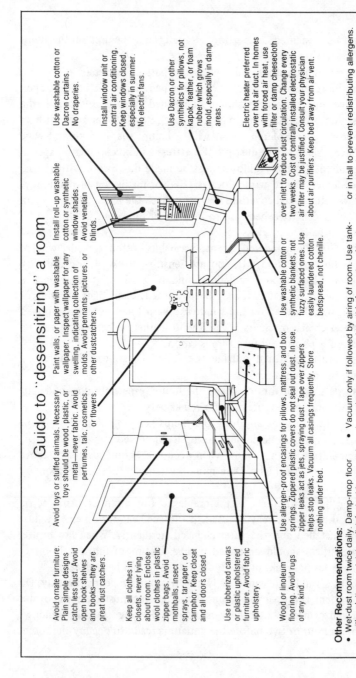

Use washable cotton or Dacron curtains. No draperies.

Install window unit or central air conditioning. Keep windows closed, especially in summer. No electric fans.

Use Dacron or other synthetics for pillows, not kapok, feather, or foam rubber which grows mold, especially in damp areas.

Electric heater preferred over hot air duct. In homes with forced air heat, use filter or damp cheesecloth over inlet to reduce dust circulation. Change every two weeks. Cost of centrally installed electrostatic air filter may be justified. Consult your physician about air purifiers. Keep bed away from air vent.

Install roll-up washable cotton or synthetic window shades. Avoid venetian blinds.

Paint walls, or paper with washable wallpaper. Inspect wallpaper for any swelling, indicating collection of molds. Avoid pennants, pictures, or other dustcatchers.

Avoid toys or stuffed animals. Necessary toys should be wood, plastic, or metal—never fabric. Avoid perfumes, talc, cosmetics, or flowers.

Use washable cotton or synthetic blankets, not fuzzy surfaced ones. Use easily laundered cotton bedspread, not chenille.

Use allergen-proof encasings for pillows, mattress, and box springs. Zippered plastic covers do not seal out dust. In use, zipper leaks act as jets, spraying dust. Tape over zippers helps stop leaks. Vacuum all casings frequently. Store nothing under bed.

Avoid ornate furniture. Plain simple designs catch less dust. Avoid open book shelves and books—they are great dust catchers.

Keep all clothes in closets, never lying about room. Enclose wool clothes in plastic zipper bags. Avoid mothballs, insect sprays, tar paper, or camphor. Keep closet and all doors closed.

Use rubberized canvas or plastic upholstered furniture. Avoid fabric upholstery.

Wood or linoleum flooring. Avoid rugs of any kind.

Other Recommendations:

- Wet-dust room twice daily. Damp-mop floor with solution containing disinfectant to prevent growth of mold spores. Oil-mop baseboards.
- Vacuum only if followed by airing of room. Use tank-type cleaner, vacuumed itself before using. Attach a second hose to outlet, placing end outside window or in hall to prevent redistributing allergens.
- No animals, birds, or reptiles in the house.
- No smoking!

Dimetane® Roomguide. Courtesy A.H. Robins Co.

Keep the doors and windows of the room closed as much as possible. Do not permit drafts and cross ventilation in this room.

Other Parts of the House

8. For house cleaning, oil mops and vacuum cleaners should be used. Do not use brooms and dusters. Keep patient out of the house while it is being cleaned. The house should be well aired before the patient returns to it after it is cleaned.

9. Upholstered furniture throughout the house and rugs should be vacuumed frequently. Daily, if possible. Whenever possible do not permit the patient to sit or lie on upholstered furniture.

10. Do not permit the use of stuffed toys. Toys should be wooden, rubber, plastic or iron. If impractical to keep patients out of a house while it is being cleaned, have them wear masks at that time.

11. Dust catchers should be removed from the house.

12. Contact with irritating odors, such as leaking stoves, refrigerators, kerosene lamps, heaters, fresh paint, camphor, tar, smoke from smudge fires, or burning trash should be avoided.

13. Be sure that all clothes and bedclothes that have been stored are well aired or cleaned before using them.

14. Patient should not handle objects that are dusty, such as books, boxes, or clothing that have been stored in cases, closets or storerooms, trunks, chests, or attics over a long period of time.

Patient should not go into attics, closets, or storerooms, or rummage in drawers.

15. Do not permit patient to wear linty materials, such as sweaters, particularly angora sweaters and knitted goods. If sweaters must be used, be sure that they have been washed or cleaned several times and most of the lint is removed.

16. Patient should not use knitting or embroidery wool.

17. Patient should never be in rooms whose temperature is below 65 degrees. Patient should never dust the erasers in school.

While the above directions may seem difficult at first, experience plus habit will make them simple, and the results will be well worth the effort.

APPENDIX C:
INHALANTS

Smoke	*Rayon*	*Kleenex*
Dust	*Fur Mix*	*Raw Silk*
Feathers		

Kapok—Is used in the stuffing of cushions, mattresses and pillows. It is also used in stuffed toys. Pillows sold under the name of silk floss are usually kapok.

Orris Root—Is used in the manufacturing of practically all scented powders, bath salts, soaps, tooth powders, cleansing creams, shaving creams, face lotions and many preparations used on the hair.

Cottonseed—Cotton fiber is used in bedding and in packing materials. The seeds are used in the manufacturing of poor grade mattresses, pillows, upholstery and toys.

Cottonseed Oil—Is used in the manufacturing of many salad oils, seasoning, and oleomargarines. Cottolene is a mixture of beef suet and cottonseed oil and is used in packing tuna, salmon, mackerel and other fish and in frying potato chips.

Karaya Gum—Is used in wave sets, dental adhesive powders, ice cream, gum drops, junkets and various tooth pastes.

Glue—Is widely used in cabinet manufacturing, bookbinding, toy animals, seals of envelopes, gelatin capsules, combs and buttons. It is derived from fish or from the hides, hoofs and bones of various animals.

Flaxseed—Is used in making linseed oil. Linseed oil is used in making linoleum, poultices, laxatives, chicken feeds, hair rinses and cattle feeds.

Pyrethrum—Is widely used in powders and sprays for the destruction of ordinary household insects. It is derived from dried chrysanthemum flowers which are members of the ragweed family; therefore these sprays and powders should not be used around patients who are sensitive to ragweed.

Cat Danders—Cat hair is used in the manufacturing of coats, carriage robes and the linings of caps, gloves and slippers as well as in the covering of toy animals and in bedding and furniture. Furs of members of the cat family such as the leopard, cougar, bob cat, tiger, and lion may also precipitate asthma.

Cow Dander—Cow hair is used in the manufacturing of animal toys. It is also used in the lining of cushions, mattresses, sofas and in chenille carpets, floor pads for rugs, and in mixing plaster and mortar.

Dog Dander—Dog hair is used in making fur coats, rugs, and robes.

Horse Dander—This may be found in blankets, stuffing of pillows, mattresses and in furniture, or in the form of clothing and draperies. It may also be carried into the environment on clothes.

Goat Dander—Goat hair is used in the manufacturing of furniture, mohair cloth, muffs, coats, various shawls (Cashmere, Indian), wigs, and oriental rugs.

Rabbit Dander—Rabbit hair is used in the manufacturing of felt. It is used in the lining of various garments such as gloves, and slippers, as well as in angora yarn, sounding hammers of pianos and the insulation of refrigerators.

Sheep Wool—Sheep wool is used in making clothing, blankets, and in other bedding.

Paints, fumes and strong odors.

APPENDIX D:
FOOD ELIMINATION DIET PROCEDURES

At the end of each initial workup, the patient is given a list of foods to avoid as much as possible and a list of foods to avoid completely.

In about 10 to 14 days the patient is asked to start adding these foods back into the diet, one at a time, along with the foods he or she is already eating. The patient should start with the food that he or she feels most necessary to resume a well-balanced diet. After choosing the food to start with, the patient is asked to eat a small amount of this food the first day and to increase the amounts gradually until this particular food has been eaten for five days. If this is a food that the patient finds difficult to eat for five days, then patient should try to eat the food for at least three days in fairly large amounts. In the case of a child, three days of trying a food is usually sufficient, as it is difficult to make a child eat some foods five days in a row. After the trial period for this food is completed, patients are asked to omit this food for two days to allow it to get out of their system. Then they may have this particular food anytime they want it, as it is apparently not a trouble-maker. Then they should go on to another food, trying it the same way.

The patient should watch for a flareup of allergy symptoms while try-ing a new food. Food allergy can affect a person in many ways; it could be wheezing, an increase in nasal congestion or postnasal drainage, headaches, vomiting, diarrhea, or skin rash. If you have a flare up of symptoms, before you blame the food, think of other things that might have brought on the symptoms, such as a visit to a home where there are dogs or cats, or being around a large number of potted plants, or a change in weather, or a visit to a dusty home, or being around where old books or newspapers have been stored and are collecting dust and molds. If there is no explanation for the symptoms, the patient is asked to stop eating the food that he or she had been trying and wait for two days before starting on a new food. In a month, the patient should go back and retry the food that was thought to have caused the flareup of symptoms. If the same flareup occurs the second time of trying this food, then the patient should avoid this food for a year before retrying it.

Patients are asked to follow through with this elimination diet, as food testing is not reliable, and the only way to tell if one has food allergies is through trying the foods and seeing which ones cause trouble.

Elimination Diet and General Rules
For Feeding An Allergic Patient

1. When a food is added to the patient's diet, the food must be eaten daily for five days. Eat a small portion the first day, and a large portion at least twice a day for the next four days.

2. Introduce one food at a time into the diet of the patient, and do not add any other food for seven days. The purpose is to see how each particular food affects the allergy, and of course if it makes it worse, it should be omitted. No new food may be considered as a part of the patient's regular diet until the trial period of five days has been observed. If the food causes no symptoms within five days of trial, it may be added to the permitted diet after eliminating two more days.

3. Add one of the foods listed to the patient's present diet every seven days.

4. Any food which causes any symptoms should be stopped promptly. Wait until the symptoms caused by the food on trial have subsided completely before trying the next food (two days).

5. It is not necessary to try any food you do not like, or do not want to add to the normal diet.

6. All foods should be thoroughly cooked before being eaten.

7. Unless you are certain of the ingredients in a certain dish, do not give it to the patient.

8. During the first year of life, only a few foods should be given.

9. When a new food is offered, it should be a single food, not mixtures. Some prepared vegetables have more than one vegetable present, and if the allergy becomes worse with the mixed foods, we would not know the single offending food.

10. Excessively large amounts of any food should be avoided. This also applies to milk.

11. No patient should be starved because of his allergy, and allowed to get into a state of malnutrition.

12. Keep a record of the effect of each food added in the chart below.

Date	Food Added	Effect

Date	Food Added	Effect

Grains

WHEAT: Wheat is mostly used in the form of white flour or whole-wheat flour. The byproducts of wheat are bran, shorts, and middlings,which are used for the food of cattle and horses. Wheat straw is used in making hats, mattresses, and mats. Coffee substitutes, such as postum, contain wheat. White flour is used in fancy sausages, toilet powders, pastes, and textiles. Wheat is contained in a great variety of prepared foods, such as the cereal preparations of infant foods. A large number of prepared flours contain wheat and other grains. Gluten is a wheat product for diabetics.

CORN: Corn is eaten mostly as corn meal or in various breakfast foods. It is usually thoroughly cooked before eating. Corn is used in the manufacture of beer and whiskey. It is used for the food of livestock and poultry, as corn starch, laundry starch, and various foods. It is mixed with other grains in various prepared flours. It is used as sizing material for textiles and wallpaper. It is also used in face and body powders and soaps. Corn is used in making soap, soap powders, oil cloth, leather substitutes, paints, and varnishes. It is used in salad oils and for shortening of bread and cakes. Mazola oil is corn oil. The byproducts of corn, such as hulls, gluten and oil cakes, are used for cattle food. The husks are often found in mattresses.

RICE: Rice is commonly eaten in the form of breakfast foods or as rice flour. As such, it is usually mixed with wheat flour and the flours of other cereals. Rice starch is used in laundries, textiles, and library paste. Rice hulls are used for fertilizer and packing materials. Rice bran is mixed with cottonseed meal for cattle food. Rice straw is used for making cattle food. The Chinese and Japanese use rice straw for making mats, robes, sandals, coats, and feeding material.

RYE: Rye is used mostly with wheat in the preparation of rye flour for rye bread. It is also made into various breakfast foods. Whiskey, vodka, and gin contain rye. It is an ingredient of paste used on labels. Rye bran is fed to cattle. Rye straw is made into braids and other straw articles such as ropes, mats, mattresses, and packing materials.

OATS: The whole kernels of oats are known as groats. The most common food preparation is oatmeal. It is mixed with wheat and other grains in prepared foods. Finely powdered oatmeal is perfumed and made into toilet articles.

BARLEY: Barley is one of the constituents of coffee substitutes. Barley meal is made into malt, beverages, and breads. Pearl barley is used in soups, puddings, cakes and breakfast foods. Barley is used in making Scotch whiskey and beer; malt sprouts and whole barley are used for cattle food.

APPENDIX E:
FOOD FAMILY RELATIONSHIPS
THAT CAN PRODUCE CROSS-REACTIVITY

Food 1	Food 2	Common Symptoms
Cola nut	Chocolate Cola drinks	Headache Rhinitis, asthma, urticaria
Legumes	Peas, beans Soybeans, peanuts The gums: acacia, karaya, tragacanth	Asthma, urticaria
Laurel	Avocado Cinnamon Bay leaf	Asthma, urticaria
Mustard	Cabbage, broccoli, cauliflower, turnips, radish, Brussels sprouts, watercress	Symptoms usually mild and varied
Poison ivy	Cashews Pistachios	Contact dermatitis, severe allergy symptoms
Fish	Various species	Urticaria, angioedema, asthma
Shellfish	Lobster Shrimp	Angioedema, urticaria, anaphylaxis

APPENDIX F:
FOODS CONTAINING SALICYLATES

Foods Containing Natural Salicylates	Foods with Added Salicylates (Flavor)
Apricots	Ice cream
Berries (blackberries, strawberries, raspberries)	Bakery goods (except bread)
Cherries	Candy
Currants	Chewing gum
Grapes (raisins, wine, wine vinegar)	Soft drinks
Nectarines	Jello
Peaches	Jam
Plums	Cake mixes
Prunes	Wintergreen flavors

Used with permission of Dr. Stephen D. Lockey, Sr.

APPENDIX G:
DO'S AND DON'T'S
TO AVOID INSECT STINGS AND BITES

1. *Do* wear shoes during the insect season.
2. *Do* wear light colors such as light green, tan, and khaki and smooth-finished fabrics.
3. *Do* shake out clothing and bedding left undisturbed for any great length of time.
4. *Do* avoid areas where stinging insects tend to frequent, such as around garbage cans, littered picnic areas, and fruit trees where fruit is rotting on the ground.
5. *Do* remove (or have removed) Hymenoptera nests, starting with search-and-destroy missions early in the spring and continue periodically until after heavy fall frosts.
6. *Do* remove insect breeding places such as ditches, old tires, barrels, cans, anywhere stagnant water can collect, and litter piles, trash, and old lumber.

1. *Don't* go barefoot or wear sandals during the insect season.
2. *Don't* wear perfume or use sweet-smelling lotions, shampoos, soaps, and the like.
3. *Don't* wear bright colors and floppy clothing, bright jewelry, suede, or leather.
4. *Don't* leave food uncovered in or out of the house.
5. *Don't*, if allergic, clip hedges, mow lawns, or pick flowers.
6. *Don't* swat if Hymenoptera are encountered. Retreat slowly, and if retreat is impossible, lie flat and cover your head with your arms.

Above all, if allergic to insect stings or bites, carry an insect-sting kit with you out-of-doors and keep one handy wherever and whenever you might encounter your nemesis.

Wear a medical warning tag or bracelet.

APPENDIX H:
DO'S AND DON'T'S OF HAND DERMATITIS

Do's

Wear heavy-duty vinyl gloves while doing chores involving contact with soap, detergent, scouring powder, or similar harsh chemicals and while handling citrus fruits, potatoes, and tomatoes.

Wear leather or heavy-duty fabric gloves when doing dry work and gardening and unlined leather gloves when outdoors in cold or windy weather.

Housewives with hand dermatitis need dishwashing machines and automatic clotheswashers. Wash hands in lukewarm water with very little soap.

All soaps are irritating. There is no "skin gentle" soap.

Don't's

Caution about contact with turpentine, paint thinner, paints, metal polish, floor polish, furniture polish, and shoe polish.

It is recommended that you remove rings when doing housework and before washing hands and do not use medicines and lubricants other than those prescribed.

Avoid rubber gloves, balsam of Peru, neomycin, gentamicin, wood alcohols, and benzocaine.

You will need to protect your hands for at least 4 months after your dermatitis has healed. There is no fast "magic" treatment for hand dermatitis. Your skin must be given a rest from irritation.

APPENDIX I:
WEATHER CHANGES AND TEMPERATURE

Hay fever and asthma are WORSE at NIGHT AND in the EARLY MORNING hours because of COOL OR COLD AIR. Whenever weather permits, you should sleep with the bedroom windows closed; at other times with as few windows open as possible. A normal individual is not affected by weather and temperature changes, but the allergic individual is affected by slight drafts, and changes in temperature and humidity; drops in temperature with attending decreases in the moisture in the air most often are responsible for symptoms. It is, therefore, advisable to have the bedroom, at least, warm during the night. A temperature between 68° and 70° F. but NOT LOWER than 65° F. should be maintained throughout the night in the bedroom. Warm, moist air is preferable to warm, dry air. A wall thermometer is a great help toward regulating the temperature in the room. Of course, if the whole house can be kept at an even temperature, it is better than if only the bedroom is so kept. Humidity of the house should be approximately 40%.

Do not stay outdoors on cold, windy days. When you are outside during cold winter months dress warmly and wear either a hat or scarf. Avoid going outside for at least one hour after bathing during cold weather. Avoid going to bed with wet hair. Upon getting out of bed wear bedroom shoes. Avoid going barefooted in the summer. Avoid wearing a wet bathing suit for prolonged period.

APPENDIX J:
SOME PHOTOSENSITIZERS

By Contact

Plants: wild parsnip, wild carrot, fig, fennel, caraway, anise, parsley, members of the Umbelliferae family, and ragweed, both pollen and plant
Insecticides which contain phenothiazine
Coal tar and derivatives in dyes, perfumes, disinfectants

Topical sulfonamides (some can produce photodermatitis, some cannot)

Antiseptic soaps and detergents that contain halogenated salicylanilides

Oil of bergamot as an ingredient in certain perfumes and toilet water

Dyes such as methylene blue, eosin, rose bengal, and acridine

Textiles, soaps, detergents, "whiter than white" products, some cosmetics containing stilbenes (hydrocarbons), some suntan lotions and some sun-screening agents

By Ingestion

Sulfonomides

Eosin used in coloring foods

Sulfonal used in sedatives

Barbiturates

By Injection

Gold

Sulfonamides

Antiseptics and medications containing acridine

Rose bengal, a dye

APPENDIX K:
SUGGESTED READING

Allergies and Your Child (Revised), D. RAPP, Coles, Toronto, 1978.

Allergy and Immunology in Childhood, F. SPEER and R.J. DOCKHORN, Eds., Charles C Thomas, Springfield, Ill., 1973.

Allergy Cooking, M. CONRAD, Thomas Y. Crowell, New York, 1960.

Allergy of the Nervous System, F. SPEER, Ed., Charles C Thomas, Springfield, Ill., 1970.

Coping With Food Allergy, C.A. FRAZIER, Quadrangle, New York, 1974.

How To Know Pollen and Spores, R.O. KAPP, Wm. C. Brown, Dubuque, Iowa, 1969.

Illustrated Genera of Imperfecti Fungi, H.L. BARNETT and D.B. HUNTER, Eds., Burgess, Minneapolis, Minn., 1972.

The Immune System (Genes, Receptors, Signals), E.E. SERCARZ, A.B. WILLIAMSON, and C.F. FOX, Eds., Academic Press, Inc., New York, 1974.

Introduction to Clinical Allergy, B.F. FEINGOLD, Charles C Thomas, Springfield, Ill., 1973.

Microbiology of the Atmosphere, 2nd ed., P.H. GREGORY, John Wiley, New York, 1973.

Parents' Guide to Allergy in Children, C.A. FRAZIER, Grosset & Dunlap, New York, 1978.

Psychosomatic Aspects of Allergy, C.A. FRAZIER, Van Nostrand, New York, 1977.

Surgery and the Allergic Patient, C.A. FRAZIER, Ed., Charles C Thomas, Springfield, Ill., 1971.

Index